TELEMEDICINE TECHNOLOGY SOLUTIONS

Author's Note

During a train ride, a lady told me how uncomfortable her diabetes-suffering 75-year-old father feels in a retirement home. He is also in the hospital more often now. I asked her why he did not stay at home with some form of telemedicine arrangement. She replied that no such set-up exists currently.

This got my attention, since I am also 75 years old, and I have since read many books and hundreds of articles about telemedicine. While the medical facets of telemedicine have been extensively described, the technical aspects are not.

The Evolution of Telemedicine Technology

Telemedicine permits doctors to evaluate, diagnose and treat patients at a distance using telecommunications technology. It is constantly evolving. Now, the technology might include a smartphone app, online video conferencing software, online diagnostics, etc. With the progress in mobile medical devices, telemedicine is incorporating sophisticated tools that can measure a patient's vitals and scan health data at home, without supervision by a medical professional.

There is a general recognition that our health care system cannot just focus on acute care. Rather, we need to focus on quality and outcome-based health care that helps manage patient and population health. It is no longer just about medicine - it is about health. The current view is that there is a need to prevent health problems, not just treat them.

Telemedicine – The Future of Healthcare

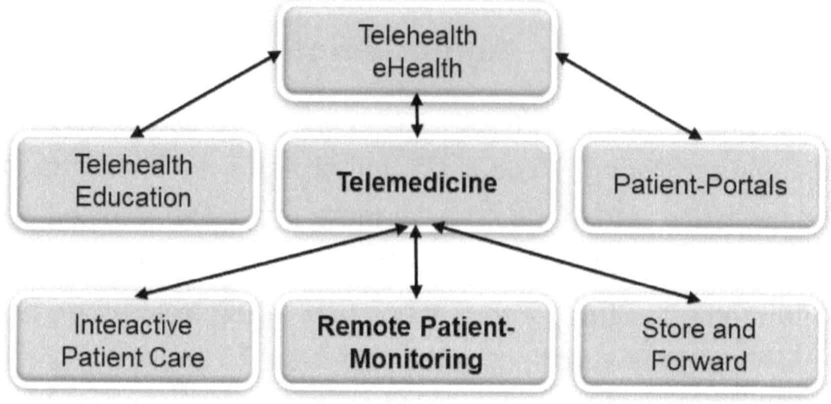

The three main parts of telemedicine include:

- Interactive Patient Care - telecommunication between physicians and patients, such as talking or examination with the help of a Smartphone w/ video.
- Patient Remote Monitoring - transmission of vital parameters, such as weight, blood pressure, oxygen saturation, glucose level, heart rate / rhythm, etc.
- Store and Forward – transfer of pictures, videos or sound. ECGs, melanoma, radiology recordings, etc.

This book is about the technology future of telemedicine; Termed sometimes also as telehealth, eHealth (electronic healthcare), mHealth (mobile healthcare), telecare, etc.

Note that most of this book consists of internet articles (the www links are clearly presented). The objective is to provide a useful framework for the technical aspects of telemedicine.

Table of Contents

Contents

Preface

The purpose of this book is to provide **information about digital technology in telemedicine** and some of the challenges associated with its implementation.

In our current healthcare system, many people are struggling to find affordable and adequate care. Costs continue to rise, and there is a growing physician shortage.

Telemedicine will be a solution that helps combat these problems. However, healthcare organizations are generally resisting changes. Although it is noteworthy that UPMC, a large US health enterprise, has recently founded a new telemedicine firm - Infectious Disease Connect (ID Connect) - to expand medical care across community clinics.

If the medical industry embraces technology and starts promoting telemedicine, the health care of the future could look very different than it does today.

Currently there is a lack of access and preparation. Training is essential. Ultimately, patients need to feel as comfortable in the virtual environment, as in a doctor's office.

While the clinical aspects of telemedicine have been studied broadly, the technical parts are not well understood. **This book focuses on the technical aspects of telemedicine.** The medical information contained in this manuscript has been derived from Internet articles.

I read many books and hundreds of articles about telemedicine before I came across the write-up "Smart Homes for Elderly Healthcare" from MDPI. It is an examination of home-based healthcare technologies. The editorial is comprehensive and illustrates the complexity of today's telemedicine technology. The R&D-focused article got my attention and inspired me to write this manuscript.

I believe that I can contribute by offering complementary business perspectives to the research-oriented article and by adding information on technologies such as artificial intelligence and new wireless networking architectures.

The existing telemedicine communication infrastructure is overloaded due to the deployment of more bandwidth-intensive connected medical and mobile devices. **Wi-Fi 6 and 5G cellular (next-generation wireless networking technologies) could be the answer.**

While telemedicine is by no means a replacement for all medical care or doctor visits, when used correctly it can be a life-enhancing solution for millions of people.

The telemedicine market is currently in a state of instability, primarily due to the flux in telecommunication technology and as a result of health insurance issues (payment problems, etc.). What's missing is a master plan for digitizing healthcare.

Although implementing telemedicine is complex and challenging, it is well worth the effort to bring care to patients who need a different type of healthcare setting.

Telemedicine improves the quality and safety of health care.

The 2019 Novel Coronavirus--2019-nCoV
(Edition II)

Health Services are monitoring the outbreak of the novel coronavirus (2019-nCoV) that was first detected in December 2019 in Wuhan City, China. Presently (end of January 2020) there are more than 11,000 confirmed cases worldwide and more than 200 deaths due to the virus. Cases have been reported in Asia, the western Pacific; Europe; the Middle East; and the United States. The virus causes mild to severe respiratory illness which can develop more serious complications like pneumonia — especially in patients that have other underlying conditions. The virus is believed to spread person-to-person via small droplets produced when an infected patient sneezes or coughs.

Telemedicine could help cope with Infectious Diseases

Innovative technologies, such as high-definition cameras, encryption software, electronic stethoscopes, microfluidic diagnostic systems, and widely available broadband Internet have expanded the potential for telemedicine. The current and future uses of telemedicine in the prevention, diagnosis, treatment, and management of infectious disease should receive more attention.

Beginning in the 1990s, early approaches to telemedicine in infectious disease focused largely on treatment of HIV/AIDS, hepatitis C, and tuberculosis. However, recent innovations allow for targeting of additional diseases and in increasingly remote settings. Telemedicine allows virtual visits between patients in the home and remote providers, permitting outpatient management of complex conditions, such as post-surgical site monitoring, and non-urgent infectious maladies, such as uncomplicated urinary tract infection. Remote provider education by videoconference and integrated clinical decision support tools create avenues to improve inpatient care, including antimicrobial stewardship. Technological strides from miniaturization of diagnostic tests to robotic telepresence physical exams improve access to infectious disease care in isolated and infrastructure-poor environments. Telemedicine in the field of infectious disease is rapidly expanding in clinical, technological, geographical, and human capacity. Recent innovations narrow gaps in access to care for populations traditionally underserved, isolated by remote geography, or lacking technological infrastructure. Future approaches will transform inpatient, outpatient, and remote care.

Novel Technologies: Essential Components of an Adequate Response to Emerging Viral Diseases

Emerging viral diseases with pandemic potential are a perpetual challenge to global health. The time-honored approach to vaccinology, which depends predominantly on isolating and growing the pathogen, has not adequately met this challenge. To effectively prepare for and respond to these continually emerging threats, it will be critical to exploit modern-day technological advances.

(Parts of the above write-up are from the JAMA Network)

Overview

By virtue of the penetration of digital devices into our daily lives, we have altered how we communicate with one another and within our social network. And we can rapidly turn to our "peripheral brain", the Google search engine, to find information or compensate for a "senior moment". This statement only scratches the surface of the way our lives have been transformed through digital innovations. Our world has forever changed.

Regrettably, we live in a time of escalating healthcare costs, and we have done almost nothing to leverage the progress of the digital era regarding healthcare. Our current system is outdated and is not using the technological developments to its full advantage.

But, the healthcare evolution advances. And for the first time in history we can digitize humans.

Digitizing a human being means formatting all of the "life codes" in a whole genome sequence. It is also about being able to remotely and continuously monitor each heartbeat, moment-to-moment blood pressure readings, the rate and depth of breathing, body temperature, oxygen concentration in the blood, glucose, brain waves activity, etc. It would not be possible were it not for the seemingly unlimited computing power via cloud server farms, biosensors, genome sequencing, imaging capabilities, and advanced health information systems.

Envisage a PC configured for telemedicine, capable of displaying all of one's vital signs in real time, sequencing parts of one's genome, or even acquiring ultrasound images of one's heart and abdomen and incorporating artificial intelligence (AI) assisted diagnosis. This embodies a technological convergence, a coalescence of distinct and far-ranging functionalities, from elemental forms of communication to the complexities of medicine.

A new era of medicine is evolving, in which each person can be almost fully defined at the individual level. We are each unique human beings, but up until now there was no way to establish one's biologic or physiologic individuality.

Putting a massive data bank to use to advance health care is expressive of the overlay of the digital and medical worlds.

But just having these technological capabilities will not advance medicine.

Governments are preoccupied with healthcare "reform," but this refers to improving access and insurance coverage and has little to do with innovation. In unison, the regulatory agencies are risk-averse and, as a result, are suppressing innovative opportunities to change healthcare.

The revolution in technology that is based on the primacy of the individual mandates also a revolution by doctors and consumers/patients in order for new healthcare to take hold.

Telemedicine Trends

A "wave" of developments forces existing healthcare delivery methods to change. These include rising medical costs, an aging population, longer life spans, and an increase in complex chronic conditions.

Technology

As previously mentioned, technology has transformed the way we go about our everyday lives. Telemedicine is a tool that can benefit anyone, regardless of age.

Fewer Family Doctors

The number of primary care physicians has steadily declined over the years, increasing the burden on practicing family care practitioners.

This limits patients' options for managing chronic diseases, minor injuries or nuisance illnesses, such as colds and flu.

Telemedicine can unburden the system.

Access to the Expertise

Medical specialists live primarily in urban areas. Telemedicine enables patients in rural areas to access those specialists. However, urban doctors may also cover multiple acute care facilities on a given day. Using telemedicine, an initial consultation can be performed to determine if a specialist needs to get in touch with the patient.

Technology Comfort

As patients become more comfortable using technology and high-speed network access is becoming more available, there are fewer barriers to using technology in order to deliver and receive medical care.

Telemedicine enables insurance companies or other providers to deliver specialty care to patients regardless of location, support chronic disease management, provide continuous monitoring of in-hospital, rural, or home-bound patients, and improve the patient experience by providing comfort, connectivity, and access to care. Patients benefit from the convenience, reduced costs and improved care.

Affordability

Telemedicine provides health care in new environments, like a patient's home, sites that are much cheaper than the emergency room or inpatient facilities. It provides a way to treat patients outside the traditional care continuum, thereby saving costs.

Chronic diseases are common in an aging population. With age, chronic diseases become more complex and frequent. Therefore, telemedicine tools, such as remote patient monitoring, provide realistic and affordable solutions that can successfully serve a population that is getting older, living longer, and is suffering from multiple, chronic complex conditions.

The Progress of Digital Technology

The amazing accomplishments, from the preparation and definition of DNA to the creation of electronic technologies that instantly and personally connect many people around the world, have triggered an unintentional digital evolution of medicine.

So far we have not had the digital infrastructure to make a big change in telemedicine. And so far, the digital revolution has barely crossed the medical world. But the emergence of potent tools to digitize human beings with full support of such infrastructure provides an unprecedented opportunity to improve the way health care is delivered. **But, continuous monitoring of physiologic data via biosensors connected to a large cohort of people will increase data flooding.**

While medicine is surprisingly resistant to change, the coming ability to digitize the biology, physiology and anatomy of each human being along with other elements - all things digital medicine - will reshape the future of medicine.

The Digital Transformation

As technology changes and improves so many different areas of life, it is only natural that these technologies also have a major impact on the healthcare sector. It goes far beyond the digitization of health records, which include comprehensive medical records, detailed patient records and private information.

The technology has made it possible to quickly identify diseases and infections, develop targeted medical solutions and offer minimally invasive surgical options. It has facilitated communication and greatly simplified the workflow.

Advanced Technology in the Healthcare Sector

Think about how technology has changed medical consultations. Remote consultations, counseling, and the immediate delivery of data such as scans, ECGs, and other reports allow patients to seek advice from super specialists or seek a second opinion virtually anywhere in the world.

Healthcare research and development has made medicines more effective and economical for patients. R&D has directed targeted treatments never before imagined. For example, we now have access to gene therapy for cancer treatment, keyhole surgery is widespread, and high-tech devices have made diagnostic processes more accurate than ever.

Artificial Intelligence (AI) in the Healthcare Sector

AI is all around us. In the medical field, it accelerates and improves diagnostic processes, creates innovative solutions and can even help with early therapeutic approaches. For example, an AI-based diagnostic device that identifies conditions such as diabetic retinopathy by scanning the retina is already a reality and has proven to be extremely accurate.

Radiotherapists and oncologists are already using AI to accelerate processes, increase accuracy, and reduce costs. Chatbots use AI-based messaging and voice systems to handle patient requests and save money. In addition, these bots can help fill in recipes, arrange appointments and speed up billing processes.

Currently, AI also plays an active role in pharmaceutical research and development: Algorithms can safely and accurately test biological or chemical interactions. This speeds up the process of bringing drugs to market; effectively saving lives. In the future, more specialists will apply artificial intelligence to diagnostic and treatment processes.

Robots in Healthcare

The idea of advanced robots performing complicated operations is no longer in the realm of science fiction. Healthcare robots are an idea whose time has come! Robotic devices that perform high-precision, minimally invasive procedures are now a reality. In addition, robots support the provision of supplements, medicines and diets that are tailored to individual patients. In the absence of human presence, robots can monitor a patient's vital signs and, if necessary, demand human intervention. They can assist in surgeries. They can help to disinfect patient rooms and reduce the exposure of humans to possible risks of infection. Robots can even perform tedious tasks such as taking blood without having to repeatedly stab the skin to find a vein. The robot can accurately identify the blood vessel and perform the extraction quickly, causing less pain.

The Internet of Medical Things (IoMT)

In healthcare, IoT (Internet of Things) becomes IoMT, bringing together health technology, telemedicine, apps and wearables. Currently, medical experts are helping with portable ECG / ECG, blood pressure, temperature and glucose monitors to prevent chronic illnesses. An estimated 60% of healthcare companies have introduced IoMT or IoT devices; contributing to increase profitability and to improve the level of care. Experts estimate that 20 to 30 billion IoMT devices will be in use by 2021.

VR/AR/MR in Healthcare

Virtual Reality, Augmented Reality and Mixed Reality are no longer limited to entertainment and games. These XR applications are changing the way physicians treat patients. They help to improve experience, reduce risk, reduce costs and offer new therapies where none existed before. For example, these applications can help children with ADHD or elderly people with Alzheimer's. Seniors with dementia, cognitive impairment, or even physical mobility problems can experience things virtually that they may not be able to do in their physical environment. XR applications can improve emotional well-being and even cognitive functions. In the future, more and more physicians will use XR applications to tailor medical procedures and make accurate diagnoses.

Blockchain and Data Science

Blockchain is a technology that uses secure, shared digital data through a peer-to-peer system and can be easily and effectively integrated into the healthcare sector. Data and health information are becoming more portable and accessible, yet remain secure and in line with industry standards. Currently, data science provides healthcare professionals with valuable information and analysis for formulating treatments.

Information on patient-drug interactions and outcomes in the patient environment may help to tailor the procedures and duration of hospital stays to allow for long-term treatment. Healthcare professionals can identify and address regional trends or epidemics, ethnic predispositions, and genetic vulnerabilities to predict and control the disease. While physicians do not yet have to implement a common technical standard for these technologies, experts predict that these technologies will become consistent and standardized in the near future.

Cloud Computing in Healthcare

In some advanced countries, submitting medical records, test results, etc. on paper is almost a thing of the past. Even digital records are now stored on the cloud rather than offline storage such as a hard drive of a medical facility. This allows healthcare professionals and patients easy access to health records. The agonizing waiting time of patients and their relatives for test results or final diagnoses is significantly reduced. The other advantage is that medical professionals on the other side of the world can quickly assess a patient's situation to offer second opinions and better, advanced treatment options.

Investing in Digital Innovation and Transformation

Digital technologies are supporting health systems' efforts to transition to new models of patient-centered care and helping develop "smart health" approaches to increase access and affordability, improve quality, and lower costs. From Blockchain, RPA, Cloud, Artificial Intelligence (AI), and Robotics, to Internet of Medical Things (IoMT), digital and Virtual Reality are just some of the ways digital technology is affecting health care.

Conclusion

The adoption and mainstreaming of digital technologies will increase. More and more of these applications are being seamlessly integrated into medicine to improve overall well-being in the coming times. These technologies will also lead to new surgical and pharmaceutical treatments, and genetic engineering will provide solutions and remedies for conditions deemed untreatable.

Data Communications

Our cohesive body functions are far more complex than this description can express, and for the most part, the systems are intact throughout our lives and function reliably to maintain our health and well-being. We take that for granted. We rarely measure the functions of our body and neither do our doctors - not because they wouldn't want to get more data, but until now that really was not possible on a continuous basis.

Once a year some individuals see a physician and get examined. Then their blood pressure is measured, the heart is listened to, and laboratory tests are done to check things like liver and kidney function, fasting blood glucose, and electrolytes.

These are random samples. But in between such occasional appointments, what is going on? What is the person's blood pressure doing during a stressful situation? How is the glucose responding to the individual's lifestyle, or how does it fluctuate during the night? Are certain foods putting undue burden on a weak pancreas to manufacture insulin? What is the heart rhythm or the level of glucose when the person feels dizzy? What is the oxygen concentration in the blood while the patient is sleeping? The list of such questions goes on and on.

The point is that today's doctor has very limited insights into the physiology of each individual.

But the field of medicine is changing. We are about to have these measurements done automatically. If there was no effort and you did not even have to remember to remove a blood pressure cuff that would make things easier.

The new healthcare technology has capabilities far beyond making things easier. Instead, the future will bring with it the ability to take continuous measurements, even during sleep and in times of significant stress. These are periods that are significant gaps in our ability to track things that are happening today.

As Healthcare Analytics put it… Healthcare Internet of Things Investment is Just Getting Started – and the devices, sensors, and clinical tools that support it – will rapidly drive new investment in a number of key market segments that will combine to create the healthcare-specific Internet of Things - from predictive analytics and ingestible sensors to home monitoring equipment and smartphone apps.

Sensors have the ability to measure every action, and as self-regulating organisms, we can fundamentally change our behavior once we receive the relevant data.

However, the proliferation of medical and mobile devices threatens to overwhelm the burden on the healthcare communications infrastructure. The next generation of wireless networking technologies could be the solution. **Wi-Fi 6 and 5G could be the turning point for healthcare networks**. 5G services were added in 2019 in some countries, and full availability of 5G is likely by 2025.

Concern About the Health Risks of Wi-Fi 6 and 5G

Concerns about Wi-Fi 6 and 5G are the latest in decades of headlines about the dangers of electromagnetic radiation. We have seen controversy over everything from the health risks of Wi-Fi to mobile phones to smart meters.

The cause of all mobile network concerns is radio frequency radiation (RFR). RFR is everything that is emitted in the electromagnetic spectrum, from microwaves to X-rays and radio waves to light from your monitor or light from the sun. Obviously, RFR is not inherently dangerous, so the problem will be to discover under what circumstances it might be a danger.

Scientists say that the most important criterion for whether a particular RFR is dangerous is whether it falls into the category of "ionizing" or "non-ionizing" radiation. Simply put, any **non-ionizing radiation is too weak to break chemical bonds**. These include ultraviolet, visible light, infrared, and anything that has a lower frequency, such as radio waves. Everyday technologies such as power lines, FM radio and WLAN fall into this area. (Microwaves are the only exception: they are non-ionizing but capable of damaging tissues; they are precise and intentionally tuned to resonate with water molecules.). Frequencies above UV, like x-rays and gamma rays, are ionizing.

Related Link: http://www.emfexplained.info/?ID=24897
https://en.wikipedia.org/wiki/Ionizing_radiation

The Electromagnetic Spectrum (EMF)

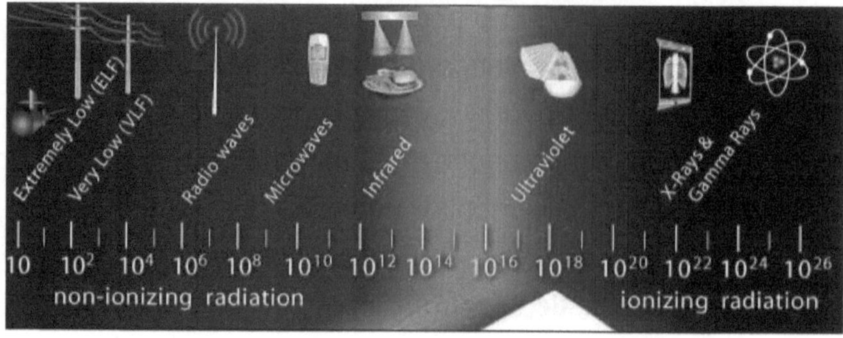

Gamma rays, X-rays, and the higher ultraviolet part of the electromagnetic spectrum are considered ionizing radiation.

In relation to EMF and health the World Health Organization (WHO) says:

"Extensive research has been conducted into possible health effects of exposure to many parts of the frequency spectrum including mobile phones and base stations. All reviews conducted so far have indicated that exposures below the limits recommended in the ICNIRP (1998) EMF guidelines, covering the full frequency range from 0-300 GHz, do not produce any known adverse health effect. However, there are gaps in knowledge still needing to be filled before better health risk assessments can be made."

WHO summary http://www.who.int/peh-emf/research/en/

5 Reasons to Trust 5G

https://www.youtube.com/watch?v=bjp2NL2n9FA

Technology Topics

The following are basic considerations for using technology to improve patient care and care coordination.

Telemedicine

From emergency care to remote patient monitoring for the management of chronic illnesses, to access to specialist care, telemedicine is changing the way health care is delivered. It extends access to routine and specialized patient care while improving patient satisfaction.

In recent years, the use of telemedicine has increased significantly. Many of the US hospitals are in contact with patients and consultants through the use of video and other technologies.

Internet Security

Cybersecurity vulnerabilities and dangers pose risks to every health care facility, and its reputation. While the increased use of network technology, Internet-enabled medical devices, and electronic databases for clinical, financial, and administrative operations, network technology, and connectivity offers significant benefits in terms of service delivery and organizational efficiency, it also increases the risk of potential cyber-security threats that require organizations to assess and manage new risks.

Interoperability

Interoperability includes the exchange and use of information within a health organization and between organizations. Obstacles to interoperability need to be addressed to support the necessary electronic exchange of health information.

EHRs - Meaningful Use

Healthcare facilities use EHRs (electronic health record) and other technologies in ways that are important to patients and communities. But the rules governing the Medicare and Medicaid EHR Incentive and Quality Payment Programs are complex and involve guidance from multiple federal agencies.

Electronic Clinical Quality Measures

eCQM (Electronic clinical quality measure) reporting must be based on information that can be collected in an automated manner, that provides valid and reliable results, and that provides an advantage that outweighs the costs.

ICD-10 and Administrative Simplification

ICD-10-CM (International Classification of Diseases, Clinical Modification) and ICD-10-PCS (Procedure Coding System) are the HIPAA (Health Insurance Portability and Accountability Act) standards for the reporting of diagnoses and procedures in hospitals. These coding systems perform an important function for payments, quality checks, benchmarking and the collection of general medical statistical data.

Telemedicine Technology

Telemedicine is changing care delivery in communities across America.

However, telemedicine, remote patient monitoring and similar technologies cannot be fully exploited due to insurance coverage, payment and other policy issues. Medicare policy is particularly challenging as it restricts the geographical and practice settings in which beneficiaries can receive services, as well as the types of services that can be provided through telemedicine and the types of technologies that can be used.

Access to broadband services and policy issues at the government level, such as licensing, also limit the ability to use telemedicine.

Systems Architecture

The development of innovative technologies has changed the way telemedicine can be practiced.

When considering the right technologies for your telemedicine program, it's important to make sure that your choices integrate easily with your existing infrastructure and are scalable to potential future applications. The right system architecture and open systems approach can lead to a nationwide delivery of telemedicine that costs only a fraction of the cost, effort, and time of second-generation (in-band) telemedicine.

Sharing Live Content is NOT Real-Time Telemedicine.

With the development of telemedicine technologies, it is no longer good enough for many medical situations to capture and share patient information. The real benefit of a clinical telemedicine encounter is that patient information can be accurately communicated between the exam site and the remote provider in real time. The use of older telemedicine technologies such as in-band telemedicine has its limitations for today's clinical needs and is more expensive than new architectural technologies.

Today's healthcare telemedicine applications typically use one of two methods of transmitting images, data and sound - either "live", in real-time transmission or store and forward transmission. While one of the two technologies is sufficient for your practice, real-time telemedicine offers many advantages over store-and-forward or content sharing applications.

Networked medical device technology

Regardless of the method of transmission, connect medical devices are a critical component of clinical telemedicine testing. Medical devices that are reliable, easy to use, and seamlessly integrated with your existing clinical workflow are the most successful.

Remote Patient Monitoring

Remote Patient Monitoring, or RPM, uses advanced technology to collect patient information outside of traditional healthcare settings. This data is then wirelessly transmitted to a healthcare facility where it is analyzed by either a computer program or a person. The data is used to identify trends or specific incidents that can reduce hospitalization and readmission by ensuring early care. Some of the types of data collected include heart rate, weight, blood pressure, blood sugar, blood oxygen levels, and electrocardiograms.

An example of the frequent use of RPM is the monitoring of falls in elderly people living at home. Sensors can either be attached to the person or to their mobility devices such as canes and walkers. The sensors can monitor location, gait, horizontal speed, and vertical acceleration to predict the likelihood of a fall and alert caregivers when the person has fallen. This information can help older people stay at home longer, while at the same time being certain that assistance will be provided when needed. RPM technology is also included in many implantable pacemakers and defibrillators so that important data can be continuously monitored. In fact, the CONNECT study (Clinical Evaluation of Remote Notification to Reduce the Time to Clinical Decision) has shown that implantable cardiac devices that actively transmit data enabled physicians to make treatment decisions 17 days earlier than those who relied on reviewing the data during in-office visits. Such RPM technologies enable physicians and individuals to better understand general health, ask specific questions and make better recommendations and treatment plans.

While with traditional RPM, data is sent periodically to a remote medical setting for analysis and assessment, a new type of RPM is evolving, with personal electronic devices that continuously transmit data. Also, with smartphone apps and connected devices, individuals can now continuously monitor many of their own personal health indicators. There are activity trackers like Fitbit and Apple Watch that record footsteps, distance traveled and heart rate. There are mattresses that monitor your sleep movement and body temperature. The scale can now be connected directly to an app to record weight and body fat over time. The apps typically include charts to show trends, make recommendations for improvement, and even provide reminders. While the data is currently used only by individuals (and also by the app company trying to sell you other things!), more and more doctors and hospitals are considering how to integrate all of that data into assessment and treatment programs, While reliability and privacy are still concerns, personal electronic devices are a great way to encourage individuals to become more involved in their own healthcare. New apps and devices are constantly being invented that can improve remote patient monitoring.

The following article offers a broad perspective.

Smart Homes for Elderly Healthcare

Excerpts from the article "Smart Homes for Elderly Healthcare - Recent Advances and Research Challenges".
https://www.mdpi.com/1424-8220/17/11/2496/htm
Published online by MDPI on **October 2017**.

Smart homes, which incorporate environmental and wearable medical sensors, actuators, and modern communication and information technologies, can enable continuous and remote monitoring of elderly health and wellbeing at a low cost. Smart homes may allow the elderly to stay in their comfortable home environments instead of expensive and limited healthcare facilities. Healthcare personnel can also keep track of the overall health condition of the elderly in real-time and provide feedback and support from distant facilities. In this paper, we have presented a comprehensive review on the state-of-the-art research and development in smart home based remote healthcare technologies.

There has been a growing awareness to develop and implement efficient and cost-effective strategies and systems in order to provide affordable yet superior healthcare and monitoring services for the people having limited access to healthcare facilities, particularly the aging population.

The elderly may require frequent, immediate medical intervention, which may otherwise result into fatal consequences. Such emergency situations can be avoided by monitoring the physiological parameters and activities of the elderly in a continuous fashion. In most emergency cases, the elderly seek in-patient care, which is very expensive and can be a serious financial burden on the patient if the hospital stay is prolonged. Remote health monitoring in a smart home platform, on the other hand, allows people to remain in their comfortable home environment rather than in expensive and limited nursing homes or hospitals, ensuring maximum independence to the occupants. Such smart homes are outfitted with unobtrusive and non-invasive environmental and physiological sensors and actuators that can facilitate remote monitoring of the home environment (such as temperature, humidity, and smoke in the home) as well as important physiological signs (such as heart rate, body temperature, blood pressure and blood oxygen level), and activities of the occupants. It can also communicate with the remote healthcare facilities and caregivers, thus allowing the healthcare personnel to keep track of the overall physiological condition of the occupants and respond, if necessary, from a distant facility.

Introduction

In recent years, the Internet-of-Things (IoT) has gained much attention from researchers, entrepreneurs, and tech giants around the globe. The IoT is an emerging technology that connects a variety of everyday devices and systems such as sensors, actuators, appliances, computers, and cellular phones, thus leading towards a highly distributed intelligent system capable of communicating with other devices and human beings. The dramatic advancements in computing and communication technologies coupled with modern low-power, low-cost sensors, actuators and electronic components have unlocked the door of ample opportunities for the IoT applications. Smart home with integrated e-health and assisted living technology is an example of an IoT application in gerontechnology that can potentially play a pivotal role in revolutionizing the healthcare system for the elderly. As the world is rapidly moving towards the new era of the IoT, a fully functional smart home is closer to reality than ever before.

In a smart home, sensors and actuators are connected through a Personal Area Network (PAN) or Wireless Sensor Network (WSN). Wearable biomedical sensors such as electrocardiogram (ECG), electromyogram (EMG), electroencephalogram (EEG), body temperature and oxygen saturation (SpO2) sensors can be connected in a Wireless Body Area Network (WBAN) or Body Sensor Network (BSN) in order to obtain automated, continuous, and real-time measurement of physiological signals. The central BSN node collects all physiological data, performs limited data processing and functions as the gateway to the PAN/WSN. The actuators operate based on the feedback from the occupants or from the central computing system. The central computing system collects environmental, physiological and activity data through the PAN/WSN, analyzes them and can send feedback to the user or activate the actuators to control appliances such as humidifier, oxygen generator, oven and air conditioner. It also functions as the central home gateway, which sends measured data to the healthcare personnel/service providers over the internet or the cellular network. In order to realize communication between all wireless sensors and actuators, standard protocols from Wireless Sensor Networks (WSNs) and ad-hoc networks are used. However, current protocols designed for WSNs are not always applicable to WBAN.

An illustration of a medical WBAN used for patient monitoring is shown in Figure 1 below. Multiple sensors can be placed over clothes or directly on the body, or implanted in tissue, which can facilitate measurement of blood pressure, heart rate, blood glucose, EEG, ECG and respiration rate.

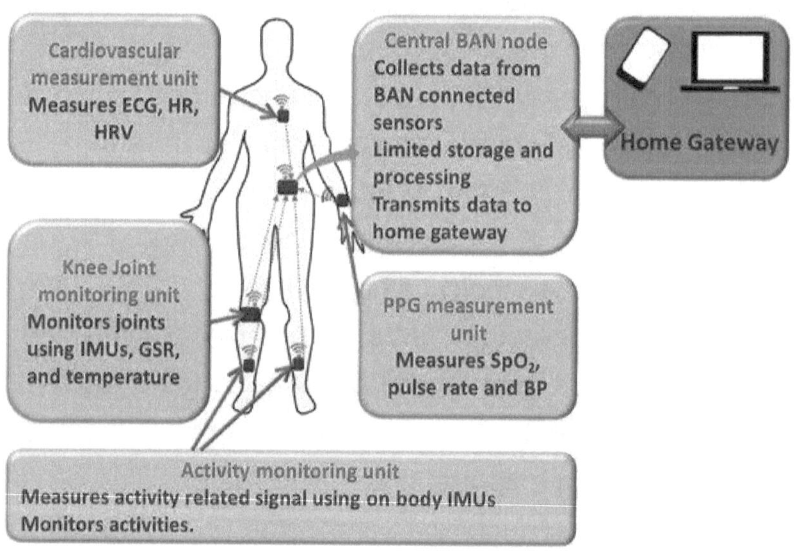

Figure 1: Wireless Body Area Network (WBAN) for wearable medical sensors

Remote Health Monitoring

E-Health and M-Health

E-health utilizes information and communication technologies to digitize and automate healthcare processes and tasks, thus enabling services like e-prescription, e-supply and e-records for patients. For example, electronic medical records (EMRs) or electronic health records (EHRs) can store and provide complete and detailed information about the medical history of patients, which can be accessed remotely and used by the authorized healthcare personnel for decision-making. Modern information and communication technologies allow continuous monitoring and recording of physiological parameters/signals, which can be stored in a central secured database. These records can be made readily available to the authorized personnel such as caregivers, emergency medical services (EMS) and family doctors when needed. A fully functional E-health system may lead towards an efficient, high quality and ubiquitous healthcare service at a lower cost and with minimal error. The infrastructure of E-health is illustrated in Figure 2.

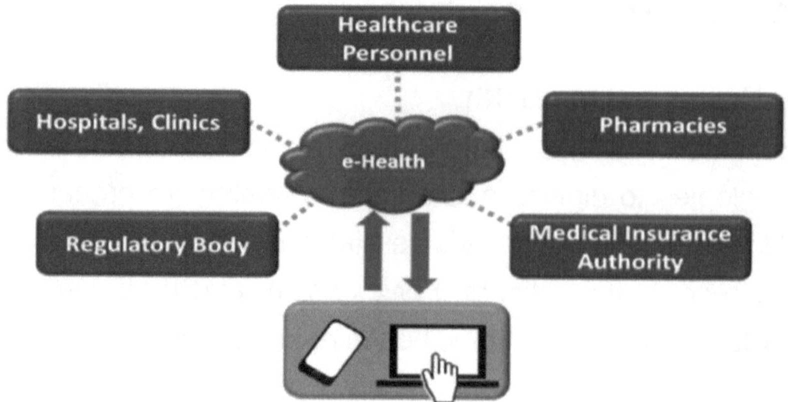

Figure 2: E-Health Infrastructure

However, the advancement of compact, portable communication and computing devices such as smartphones, and tablets has created the pathways for the evolution of M-health from the classical E-health concept. M-health is based-on modern mobile communication technologies such as Enhanced Data GSM Environment (EDGE), 3G, High Speed Packet Access (HSPA), and Long-Term Evolution (LTE), which offer high-speed and seamless data transfer from anywhere, at any time, thus allowing people to remain connected with the central M-health system.

As mentioned earlier, a network of environmental, biomedical, and motion sensors, which can measure and send measured data to the remote facilities through the gateway, can be deployed at home. Wearable biomedical sensors located in (implanted devices, e.g., pacemaker, insulin injector), on (e.g., ECG or EEG electrodes), or around (e.g., gesture detectors, external devices) the human body can be connected in a BAN, thereby enabling ubiquitous, unobtrusive continuous health monitoring. The data collected by the sensors are transmitted to a central BAN node, which can process and transfer information to an external device (the user's mobile phone) or a remote workstation (a nurse station in a hospital or nursing home). Monitoring of key parameters such as patient's activity, heart rate (HR), blood pressure (BP), respiration rate (RR) and body temperature (BT) from a remote station and sending feedback accordingly over the M-health system may potentially lead towards the E-ambulatory care system.

It is expected that modern miniature sensing and actuating technologies along with the advanced connectivity platforms such as BAN and home based WSN as well as increased penetration of high-speed internet globally will play a pivotal role in moving towards the home-based remote healthcare services from the conventional in-clinic care. The network of sensors monitors the condition of the subject under supervision and sends the information to a distant healthcare facility over the internet or it can automatically call for EMS in case of an emergency. However, ensuring seamless connectivity, secured transmission channels and data storage are the key challenges in developing a complete infrastructure of an E-health or M-health system for medical information management and continuous monitoring of health. Moreover, interoperability among different protocols and standards is also critical for the consistent operation of the system. In addition, precise and accurate measurements of key health parameters are vital for a reliable health monitoring system.

Home-Based Remote Health Monitoring

The advancement of miniaturized and inexpensive sensors, embedded computing devices, and wireless networking technologies paved the way for realizing remote health monitoring systems. Remote health monitoring allows un-obtrusive, ubiquitous, and real-time monitoring of physiological signs without interrupting the daily activities of individuals. People can remain in their familiar home environment and enjoy their normal lives with the friends and family while their health is being monitored and analyzed from a remote facility based on the physiological data collected by different on-body sensors. The system can perform long-term health trend analysis, detect anomalies, and generate alert signals in the case of an emergency.

In order to facilitate continuous monitoring of health, various E-health devices are proposed in the literature. EnViBo, which stands for embedded network for vital sign and biomedical signal monitoring, is such a platform for the ambulatory monitoring of adults with medical conditions or people working under extreme conditions such as firefighters and rescue personnel. An open-source platform for a wireless body sensor network named DexterNet was introduced. This platform comprises a body sensor layer (BSL), a personal network layer (PNL), and a global network layer (GNL) that supports real-time and persistent human monitoring in both indoor and outdoor environments.

Telemedicine is an advanced form of E-health service which provides remote healthcare support, analyzes the trends in medicine usage and makes the information available to the authorized personnel with the help of modern communication technologies, thus allowing faster and affordable healthcare services. In a recent study on the effectiveness of telemedicine, it was found that telemedicine was beneficial to reduce mortality due to different causes. Telemedicine also effectively reduces hospital admission, length of stay and mortality due to heart failure. Telemedicine systems for in-home monitoring of vital signs exist. The sensors communicate with an android based smartphone using Bluetooth. The smartphone functions as the gateway to a long range communication network such as a 3G cellular phone network or wireless local area network (WLAN). A tele-medicine system that can measure several physiological signs of the resident and send them to a computing platform for further analysis was also developed. The medical staffs can keep track of the signs over a web-based interface. The system is capable of transmitting real-time information to a remote medical server over both the cellular networks and internet in case of an emergency or on request. Some technology companies are currently offering tele-medicine services over web-based platform. The services include secure video communication between doctor and patients, remote health monitoring, and emergency care service.

Intelligent furniture such as smart chairs and smart beds can also be utilized for measuring physiological data at home. For example, a smart bed can monitor the health status and sleep patterns of an individual. It can also be used to detect a heart attack of the cardiac patients while they are on the bed or sleeping. The system can immediately inform the central system, caregivers, EMS or any authorized personnel in an automatic fashion, thus reducing the risk of fatality.

Internet-of-Things and Connected Homes

The developments of low-power wireless communication technologies, miniaturized sensors and actuators as well as growing penetration of internet, tablets, and smartphones are leading us towards the new era of the IoT. Connected homes or smart homes use the concept of the IoT, which offers a platform to monitor safety and security of the home or to automatically control the home environment or appliances, over the internet from anywhere. The IoT can be defined as a network of intelligent objects that is capable of organizing and sharing information, data and resources, decision making, and responding to feedback. It allows human-to-human, human-to-things and things-to-things interaction by providing a unique identity to each and every object. The US National Intelligence Council (NIC) considered the IoT technology as one of the six disruptive civil technologies that can potentially impact US national power. Some researchers envisioned the IoT as an emerging field that can enable new ways of living by bridging the physical world with the digital computing platform by means of smart sensing and actuating devices, and appropriate communication technologies such as Bluetooth Low Energy (BLE), ZigBee and ANT. Therefore, the concept of IoT can be exploited in a wide range of applications (Figure 3) such as E-health, assisted living, enhanced learning, intelligent transportation, environmental protection, government work, public security, smart homes, intelligent fire control, industrial monitoring and automation.

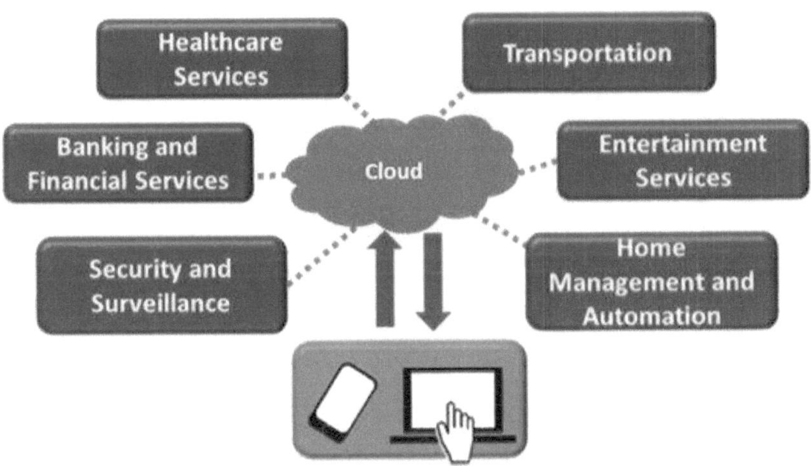

Figure 3: Applications of the Internet of Things (IoT).

Traditional homes, in spite of being energy-hungry, are generally not designed to monitor the environment of the home, or physiological conditions and activities of the occupants by itself. A smart home, in contrast, is a traditional house embedded with smart devices and modern communication technologies that can facilitate remote and automatic monitoring of home environment, security and overall health status of the occupants. However, in order to achieve widespread acceptance among the users, smart homes need to be affordable. Therefore, low-power and efficient communication technologies and public networks, along with low-cost devices are critical for smart homes. In addition, several key technological challenges such as full interoperability among the interconnected devices, high degree of precision and accuracy, processing resource limitation, and privacy and information security need to be addressed. A successful implementation and penetration of fully-fledged smart homes may lead towards smart cities or intelligent residential districts in the near future.

Layered Architecture of a Smart Home

Smart homes may include a set of environmental, activity and physiological sensors, actuators connected through a wireless communication medium. The advancement in low-power, smaller dimension sensing, actuating and transceiver systems coupled with modern communication technologies and inexpensive computing platforms such as field programmable gate array (FPGA), microcontrollers, microprocessors paved the way for low-cost smart home systems.

A four-layer architecture for smart home is presented as follows:

Layer 4 – Services

- Telemedicine and Healthcare Services
- Safety and Emergency Services
- Long-term Remote Monitoring Support

Layer 3 – Computing and Decision Making Platform

- Information Analysis
- Context-based Learning
- Prediction by Intelligent Reasoning
- Decision Making and Alert Notification

Layer 2 - Communication Network

- Secured Communication Channels
- Bridge Physical and Computing Platforms
- Sensors and Appliances Discovery

Layer 1 – Sensors and Actuators

- Environmental Sensors
- Wearable Sensors for Health Monitoring
- Actuators for Appliance Control

Sensors and Actuators

Sensors and actuators play the key role in smart home by bridging the gap between the physical world and the digital domain. Smart homes use several sensors to collect data about the home environment such as light illumination level, temperature, pressure, gas leakage, oxygen level, and about the activity or location of the occupants by using inertial measurement units, RFID tags or passive infrared (PIR) sensors. Physiological parameters such as BP, HR, SpO2, galvanic skin response (GSR), RR can be measured using wearable sensors. Actuators can respond to the feedback from the occupants or from the central decision making platform by performing small scale maneuver to control environment or to deliver drugs such as insulin on occupant's body. These sensors and actuators can communicate with the central computing and decision making platform over the wireless communication medium. The sensors, particularly the wearable medical sensors need to be energy efficient and unobtrusive in order to facilitate long-term monitoring. Sensors and actuators with embedded energy harvesting technologies can effectively increase the running time of the ambulatory devices.

Communication Network

All sensors and actuators in the smart home are connected with the central communication and decision making platform though a communication network, which forms the second layer of the smart home architecture. All physiological and environmental signals measured by the sensors are transmitted to the central computing node over a wireless and/or wired communication medium. Although wired connection is a feasible solution for fixed-position based environmental sensors, it is not suitable for wearable and long-term monitoring systems. Wired connections for the wearable BSN may cause inconvenience to the user and restrict users' mobility. It may also cause occasional connection failure among the on-body sensors. Textile based conductive medium such as conductive fabrics can be used to communicate with the on-body sensors as an alternative to the wired connection. Conductive fabrics can be produced using conventional textile technologies such as weaving, stitching, embroidery, and screen printing. However, conductive textiles suffer from low durability and limited washability, thus resulting in poor or failed connectivity after prolonged use. Therefore, modern low-power wireless communication technologies appear to be the most viable and reliable medium for short-range communication. Table 2 presents the key features of some commonly used wireless technologies for short range communication.

The wearable medical sensors can be connected in a BSN, where the central BSN node is connected with all environmental sensors and actuators through the WSN. All the sensors and actuators in the smart home are connected to form a Local Area Network (LAN) or Personal Area Networks (PAN) and to provide data communication inside the smart home. The central decision making platform can communicate with any sensors and actuators in the network using the WSN to collect data or send feedback to perform necessary actions, if required.

Wireless Tech.	Frequency	Range	Data Rate	Power (mW)	Maximum Nodes	Network Topologies	Security
RFID	13.56 MHz 860–960 MHz	0–3 m	640 kbps	200	1 at a time	peer-to-peer (P2P) passive	N/A
Bluetooth	2.4–2.5 GHz	1–100 m	1–3 Mbps	2.5–100	1 M + 7 S	P2P, star	56–128 bit key
BLE	2.4–2.5 GHz	1–100 m	1 Mbps	10	1 M + 7 S	P2P, star	128-bit AES
HomePlug GP	1.8–30 MHz	~100 m	4–10 Mbps	500	-	P2P, star, tree and mesh	128-bit AES
EnOcean	902, 928, 868 MHz	30–300 m	125 kbps	~0.05 with energy harvesting	-	P2P, star, tree and mesh	128-bit AES
ZigBee	2.4–2.5 GHz	10–100 m	250 kbps	50	65,533	P2P, star, tree and mesh	128-bit AES
WiFi	2.4–2.5 GHz	150–200 m	54 Mbps	1000	255	P2P, star	WEP,WPA, WPA2
DASH7	315–915 MHz	200 m–2 km	167 kbps	<1	-	P2P, star, tree and mesh	128-bit AES
Insteon	RF: 869.85, 915, 921 MHz powerline: 131.65 KHz	40–50 m	38 kbps (RF) 2–13 kbps (powerline)	-	64,000 nodes per network	P2P, star, tree and mesh	256-bit AES
Sigfox	868/902 MHz	10–50 km	10–1000 bps	0.01–100	-	P2P, star	No default encryption
NFC	13.56 MHz	5 cm	424 kbps	15	1 at a time	P2P	AES
Wireless HART™	2.4 GHz	50–100 m		10	-	P2P, star, tree and mesh	128-bit AES
6LoWPAN	2.4 GHz	25–50 m	250 kbps	2.23	-	P2P, star, tree and mesh	128-bit AES
ANT	2.4–2.5 GHz	30 m	20–60 kbps	0.01–1	65,533 in one channel	P2P, star, tree and mesh	64-bit key
Z-Wave	860–960 MHz	100 m	9.6–100 kbps	100	232	mesh	128-bit AES

AES: Advanced Encryption Standard.

Table 2: Communication technologies for smart homes

Computing and Decision Making Platform

The third layer of smart home architecture is responsible for computing and decision making, thus functioning as the brain of the system. This layer is equipped with computing system such as smartphone, computer or custom-built processing node based on Field Programmable Gate Array (FPGA) or microprocessors. It gathers data from the sensors and actuators over the WSN, processes, and analyzes measured data, and sends feedback to the user or to the actuators. It may also store measured data, display the results to the user, and may run prediction algorithms. The prediction algorithms can exploit the features of artificial intelligence (AI) and make use of deep learning and machine learning techniques such as artificial neural network (ANN), support vector machine (SVM), and K-Nearest Neighbors (KNN) to learn and develop models for the home environment as well as for the behavioral and physiological patterns of the occupants. Researchers from the University of Missouri, Columbia equipped an independent senior living facility, called TigerPlace, with smart sensors to monitor and assess the residents' activity and overall health. A wide variety of sensors were installed to monitor occupants' daily activities, pulse and respiration. The researchers, however, initially developed a fuzzy-logic based model that can produce linguistic summaries of two activities—movements in bed and movements in the apartment—by analyzing the motion sensor data collected over a longer period of time. The work may be further extended to incorporate more sensor data and detect anomalies by assessing the magnitude of deviations from the normal patterns in the activities and physiological data.

Such models are used by the computing platform to make predictive decisions about the home environment or occupant's health status based on the information received from several sensors. The adoption of AI will also allow this platform to exploit robotics to control the smart home peripherals and to provide services to the occupants in an automatic fashion with continuous improvements in accuracy and precision over time. One such platform, Lab-of-Things

(LoT) is developed by Microsoft Research that uses an operating system named HomeOS to monitor, manage, and control interconnected devices in homes and analyze data received from the sensors. This layer is also responsible for ensuring a secured, long-range communication channel to the remote service provider. It can transmit the measured data, key physiological or environmental parameters over the internet or cellular network, thus functioning as the home gateway to the remote facility. This platform monitors and assesses the measured physiological or environmental data continuously. If any abnormality in the home environment or in the vital signs of the user's health is detected, it can raise an alarm or send alert messages to the service providers in the form of voice call, text message or e-mail.

Services

The top layer of the smart home architecture consists of the services delivered to the user by the service providers. These services may be associated with the health of the occupants, environment, safety, or security of the home and the residents. Services provided to the smart home can be tailored according to the requirements of the occupants based on the level of medical attention or safety and security required. In a smart home, the gateway platform functions as the primary service provider, for example, by activating necessary actuators to control the home environment, door locks or dosage, in the case of automated drug delivery. The gateway system may adopt AI technologies to assess the safety, security and environment of the home and control the smart devices to provide the occupants with better services. The gateway can learn and keep continuous track of the occupants' physiological conditions with the help of the BSN-connected wearable health sensors. The AI technologies implemented in the gateway will allow the smart devices in the smart home to be controlled to adjust the home environment according to the occupants' requirement. It can also monitor the home environment and can detect any hazardous situation such as presence of smoke or gas leakage using the environmental sensors installed at different places in the home. In case of any anomalous physiological or environmental conditions, the gateway raises alarms and sends electronic notifications such as emails, text messages, and phone calls to the secondary service provider.

The secondary service provider is **the central hub** of all the subscribed smart homes and responsible for management, maintenance, connectivity, and information security of the smart home network and systems. **It continuously monitors for alarms or emergencies and immediately notifies other third party services such as emergency medical service (EMS), caregivers, police station and fire station, if necessary**.

Interoperability and Standardization

One of the key concerns in adopting the IoT technologies for smart homes evolves from the fragmentation of the technologies. The fragmentation of the IoT technologies, which is not only driven by technology constraints but marketing and business policies also causes lack of interoperability among the smart devices, platforms and systems. These issues need to be addressed for ubiquitous adoption of the IoT in smart homes. Smart homes, as the term implies, are envisioned to be fully automated, energy efficient, and sustainable as well as capable of monitoring, assessing the health, safety and wellbeing of the occupants. It also requires a robust communication platform and might also facilitate assistance to the occupants for the ADLs. Therefore, the smart homes are expected to be equipped with a wide variety of devices, systems and platforms from different suppliers in order to provide the occupants with a wide range of services. However, the communication technologies used in those devices and systems may vary from supplier to supplier, thus leaving a fragmented IoT market and thereby posing a great challenge for the smart home service providers in bringing together different technologies in a cost-effective and energy-efficient manner. For example, there exists long-range cellular communication technologies such as GSM, EDGE, 3G, HSPA, and LTE along with several non-cellular short or medium range wireless connectivity solutions presented in Figure 5, while new technologies such as ABB-free@home® and Thread Protocol are emerging. Each of these non-cellular technologies offer its own advantages and also has its limitations. However, the key concern evolves from the fact that they often are not compatible with each other.

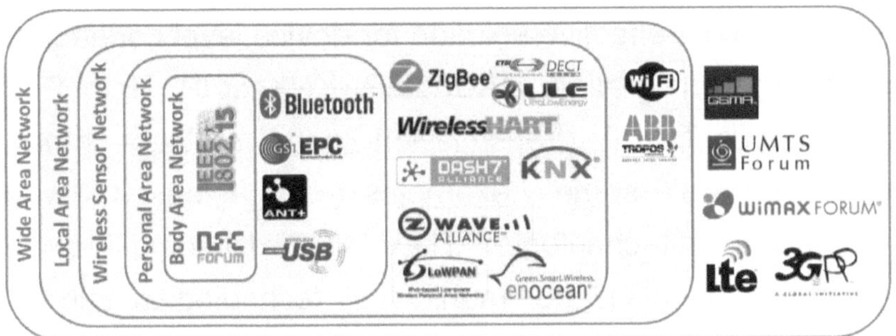

Figure 5: Fragmentation of wireless communication platforms.

A common, extensible and standardized platform is thus required to ease the integration of different technologies, systems and services from different manufacturers. The internet of things, services and people (IoTSP) is such a platform that is particularly designed for building automation. In fact, there exists a number of standards for the IoT developed by major standard development organizations (SDOs) such as Institute of Electrical and Electronics Engineers (IEEE), International Organization for Standardization/International Electrotechnical Commission (ISO/IEC), International Telegraph Union-Telecommunication Standardization Sector (ITU-T), Internet Engineering Task Force (IETF), and European Telecommunications Standards Institute (ETSI). Each SDO has their own point-of-view towards the IoT; however they are putting their efforts to bridge the gap among the standards. The interoperability issue is currently being addressed by adopting the internet protocol (IP) as the common platform, which, by assigning local IP addresses for the devices and systems, allows for realizing a cost-effective solution for device level connectivity and system integration. BACnet/IP, KNXnet/IP, HomePlug, and Modbus TCP/IP (transmission control protocol /internet protocol) are some examples of IP-based wired communication technologies. There also exist some IP-based versions of wireless communication technologies such as IPv6 over Low-Power Wireless Personal Area Networks (6LoWPAN) over Bluetooth, ZigBee IP, 6LoWPAN over DECT ULE, and Thread.

In addition, there is a growing consensus among the engineering and scientific community of using Representational State Transfer or RESTful web services to develop the application programming interfaces (APIs) for the IoT applications. RESTful web services are light weight and highly flexible, which uses Hypertext Transfer Protocol (HTTP) for data communication. It allows the system to communicate with different devices in the network running on different communication platforms. It thus allows for building a bridging platform for all the sensors, actuators and systems used in the smart home, irrespective of the manufacturer and can successfully fulfill the integration requirements, which are critical for seamless operation of the smart home. The adoption of RESTful web services in the IoT may also enable adopting other semantic technologies such as OPC UA (Open Platform Communications Unified Architecture) and oBIX (Open Building Information Xchange) from the internet industry in future.

Smart Monitoring Systems for Elderly and for People with Disability

As people age, often, their need for medical support grows, which may result in frequent and unplanned medical attention or in-clinic healthcare services. In order to get long term healthcare service, some elderly people need to stay in long term care (LTC) centers, which are expensive as well as of limited capacity. However, the ongoing development towards the IoT technology can play a pivotal role for the growth of elderly healthcare systems. In a smart home, various key physiological signs of the elderly can be measured and monitored using simple, low-cost sensors from a remote healthcare service center over a secured communication platform, thus offering a cost-effective solution for long-term health monitoring. This will also allow the elderly to lead an independent life in their homes while ensuring maximum comfort, safety and security. An illustration of a smart home solution used for elderly people is shown in Figure 6.

The smart homes can benefit from artificial intelligence (AI), which can gather and analyze information regarding the occupant's activities and health status, identify and report any anomalies. The AI system includes a database that stores residents' behavioral and physiological patterns, and medical histories. In case of a medical emergency, this system can raise an alarm and share medical profiles with the concerned authority over a secured channel, thus allowing the residents to have immediate and appropriate medical attention.

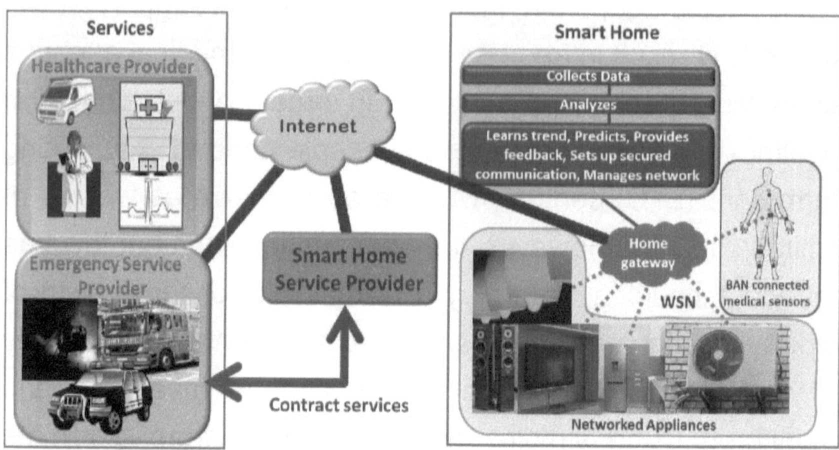

Figure 6: Schematic diagram of a smart home showing the network among different stakeholders.

Recently, a wide range of wearable systems have been proposed for elderly healthcare that can monitor vital signs as well as the activities of the patients. These systems include sensors software and wireless technology to collect, process, analyze and transfer physiological and activity related data to a remote healthcare center. Intelligent homes may incorporate BAN connected wearable systems as well as environmental sensors, actuators, and cameras, all connected through a WSN.

Automated Emergency Call Systems

Some smart home solutions monitor the environment of the home as well as the physiological parameters of the elderly and can communicate with service providers in case of an emergency. The Allocation and Group Awareness Pervasive Environment (AGAPE) is such a healthcare system designed for patients living far from a healthcare facility. When the AGAPE detects any anomalies in the data measured by the on-body sensors, it starts looking for and contact nearby caregiver groups. Once the group is informed, AGAPE locates the patient's profile and forwards it to them. Meanwhile, AGAPE contacts and keeps other groups informed about the situation and requests additional assistance, if necessary.

Automated Activity and Fall Detection Systems

Smart homes need to distinguish between normal and abnormal activities with high accuracy in order to respond with appropriate actions. Some smart homes use video-based systems to monitor and recognize different activities. Although these systems can recognize complex gait activities, they restrict the user to reside within a specific area. In addition, these systems are expensive and require high processing resources. Motion sensors such as accelerometers, gyroscopes and magnetometers, in contrast, are smaller, simple to use and low-power devices, thereby suitable for monitoring human activities in a wearable platform. These motion sensors along with vital signs sensors can be embedded in socks, armbands, t-shirts in order to receive comprehensive information about the overall health status of the subjects. Other motion detectors such as passive infrared sensors (PIR) can be used to detect the location of the subjects in the house.

Falls are one of the leading causes of injuries and death among the elderly. In case of non-injurious falls, around 47% of persons experiencing a fall need external support to get up. A general representation of fall detection system is shown in Figure 7. When the system detects a fall, it will inform the corresponding personnel by triggering an alarm.

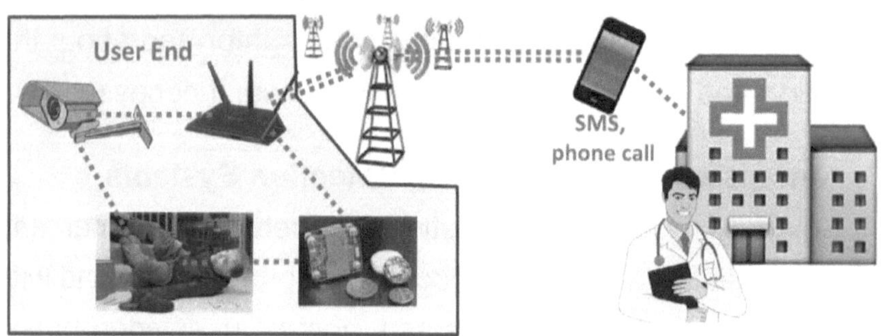

Figure 7: Remote fall detection system.

Vital Signs Monitoring Systems

Vital signs, which include heart rate (HR), body temperature (BT), respiration rate (RR) and blood pressure (BP), are the most basic parameters that are routinely monitored by the medical professionals to get a good overview about the health of the patients. Several vital signs monitoring systems are reported in the following article - **"Wearable Sensors for Remote Health Monitoring"**

Reminding Systems

Memory and cognitive function in the older adults decline gradually with age causing many elderly people to suffer from severe memory loss and dementia. This loss of cognitive functionality can disrupt their daily living and even be dangerous at times, for example, if a person forgets to take the medicine or takes higher doses than prescribed. Therefore, a reminding system would be very useful for the elderly in their daily life. The system raises an alert signal at a pre-scheduled time and can send detailed information to the user or the caregivers, as needed.

Wedjat is such an application that is designed to remind the individuals about their medicines as well as meals. The application takes the prescription as the input and reminds the patient to take the medicine about 1 to 15 min before the scheduled time, provides in-take directions and keeps records of all taken and missed medicines.

An activity tracking application in android platform for smart homes was presented (14th International Conference on Advanced Communication Technology, PyeongChang, Korea). The system has a reminder application for the elderly and a separate application for the caregivers or the family members of the elderly. The application reminds the elderly about medicines, and scheduled tasks. It also notifies the caregivers or family members for assistance in case of critical situations.

A hardware based medication reminder system is proposed (2016 IEEE International Conference on Systems,

Man, and Cybernetics, Budapest, Hungary). This system reminds the patient about the medicine at a prescheduled time, provides them with appropriate dose of medicine, and gives vocal guidance about the in-take procedure. The system uses sensors and actuators to monitor the patient's activities and control the medicine dispensing units with right amount of dose. It also can facilitate communication with the caregivers if necessary.

Automated Health Assessment

The automatic and continuous assessment of the cognitive and physical health of the residents is one of the key services that the smart monitoring systems can facilitate. Continuous monitoring and real time assessment of health can be useful in balance and fall analysis, rehabilitation following an injury, and can also enable early detection of physical and cognitive impairment. For example, gait patterns tend to differ from its normal behavior at the early onset of some neurodegenerative diseases, such as Alzheimer's and Parkinson's. A person at the primary phase of Parkinson's tends to make small and shuffled steps, and may also experience difficulties in performing key walking events, such as starting, stopping, and turning. Therefore, quantitative assessment of daily activities, gait patterns, and vital signs can be very useful for early detection of a potential health problem.

The smart monitoring systems can integrate automated activity monitoring and vital sign monitoring systems to evaluate the overall health status of the residents with the help of modern machine learning techniques. The automated assessment algorithm generally begins with the extraction of key parameters/features from the sensor data associated with a particular activity or physical health.

These features are then used by an appropriate machine learning algorithm to make quantitative assessment about the overall health status.

Smart Homes for Elderly Healthcare: Prototypes and Commercial Solutions

In the above discussion, we have presented different healthcare and monitoring systems reported in the literature. As depicted in Figure 9, a fully-fledged smart home requires all such systems along with a wide range of physiological and environmental sensors to be integrated in a common platform that poses new challenges in terms of volume of information, uninterrupted connectivity, interoperability, and most importantly, privacy and data security.

Many researchers along with some technology companies around the world have been working to overcome these technological challenges. In this section, we present some prototypes of smart homes reported recently in the literature. We also discuss some commercial smart-home solutions currently available in the market.

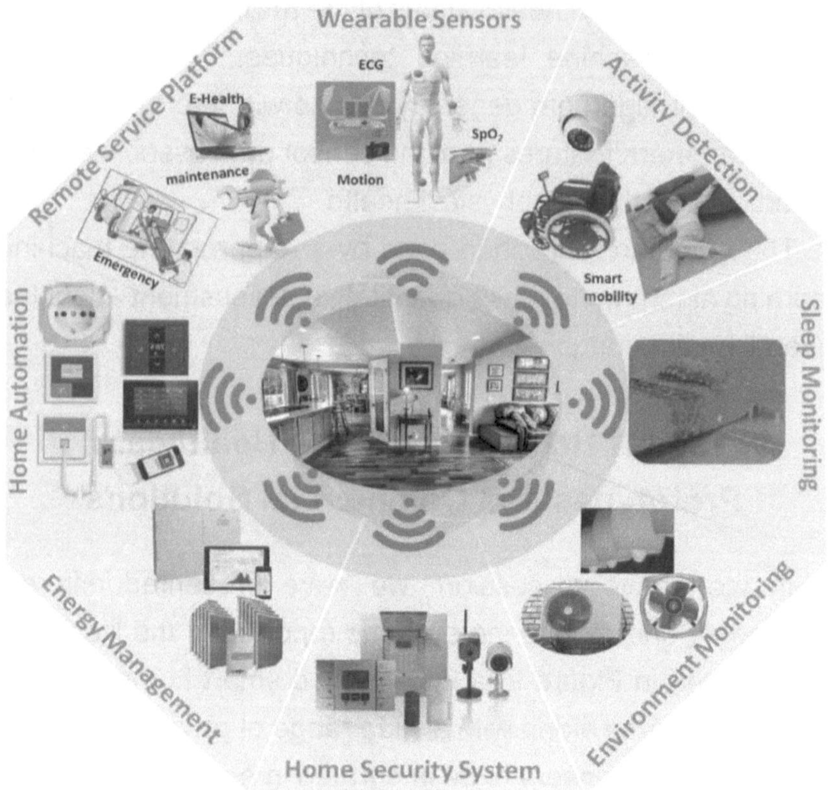

Figure 9: Smart homes integrated with automated systems for elderly healthcare

Smart Home Solutions in the Literature

The University of Colorado, Boulder in one of the earliest smart home projects, explored the concept of a self-automated home. The researchers developed a prototype that is capable of monitoring and controlling the temperature, water, ventilation system and lighting in the home. The researchers exploited neural networks to learn and predict the behavioral patterns from the lifestyle of the residents and to accommodate the needs of the occupants accordingly.

A smart home system, MavHome (Managing An intelligent Versatile Home) was introduced, that used several sensors to perceive and analyze home environment as well as the residents' action. The MavHome intelligent agent learns the patterns observed in the residents' activities and developed a statistical model to make predications and control the home environment accordingly.

Researchers at University of Florida, Gainesville developed a programmable pervasive computing space for the smart home (GatorTech Smart House) that allows automatic integration of system components. They developed an extensible and easy-to-integrate service framework, which contains service definitions for all system components, thus enabling automatic discovery and integration of the components. The system uses a multi-layered architecture to discover and communicate with the sensors and actuators. The architecture also facilitates analysis of sensory data and contextual information to provide an intelligent assistive living environment for the occupants. One may find other early implementations of smart homes which includes the 'Intelligent Workplace' at Carnegie Mellon University, Georgia Tech Aware Home, Smart Medical Home at University of Rochester, and MIT intelligent room project.

Researchers from Carleton University, Ottawa presented an overview of smart home system for monitoring the elderly health and wellbeing. They developed an initial prototype of smart home by installing and integrating several sensors such as magnetic switches, infrared motion sensors and pressure sensitive mats to monitor the home environment and security. They proposed a four-tier alarm system based-on the severity of the detected anomalies. Another group of researchers from the same and other universities studied the feasibility of integrating the IoT with web-based services and cloud computing. They installed actuators to control lights and fans as well as several sensors such as temperature, humidity, ambient light and proximity sensors to monitor home environment. All sensors and actuators were connected over the ZigBee protocol and can be monitored or controlled over a cloud-based computing service.

A design and implementation of a mobile healthcare system (mHealth), particularly for wheelchair users was presented (2014, IEEE 18th CSCWD, Hsinchu, Taiwan). Several environmental sensors, actuators for appliance control and cameras were installed in a 6 m × 6 m room. The user wore a HR sensor as well as an ECG sensor, which facilitate cardiovascular activity measurement. A wireless pressure cushion and accelerometer were installed in the wheelchair to detect the falls and for activity monitoring. The researchers also developed an Android-based software interface to monitor and display the physiological signs as well as to control the home environment by activating the actuators. The software collaborates with a third-party service to send text messages & voice calls in case of an emergency.

An advanced platform for in-house health monitoring and assessment called The ORCATECH Life Laboratory was developed by the Oregon Center for Aging and Technology (ORCATECH). The researchers mostly exploited commercial ambient and passive wireless sensors to monitor and assess the physical and cognitive health of the occupants. The sensors were connected to a wall-mounted hub, which functioned as the gateway of the smart home and was able to transmit the measured data to a cloud-based server over the internet or 3G mobile communication protocols. The computing and decision making layer was implemented in the server, which processed and analyzed the sensor data and ran advanced machine learning algorithms to assess occupants' overall health status based on several parameters such as walking speed, sleep quality, and activity.

A WSN-based smart home, designed for elderly health care was proposed (2015, ICNTE, Navi Mumbai, India). The smart home comprises a set of wireless sensors, which facilitates monitoring the temperature and safety of the home. The system used ZigBee technology for implementing the WSN and was capable of raising an alarm in case of an emergency.

A smart home platform (Springer: Berlin, Germany, 2016) was developed primarily for monitoring home environment and residents' activities. The system deployed cameras and wearable inertial measurement unit (IMU) to measure and assess movement patterns. All sensors were connected over the Bluetooth Low Energy (BLE) and IEEE 80 2.15.4 platform, whereas the gateway, video camera and computers were connected over the Wi-Fi. The gateway supports both IEEE 80 2.15.4 and Wi-Fi and functions as the hub for all sensors, and computers in the home. It also can communicate with a remote data hub through a virtual private network (VPN).

A prototype of a smart home (Pilot SMARTA Project, Gerontology 2017) was capable of monitoring several physiological signs such as ECG, BP, SpO2, and BT along with few environmental parameters and appliances. The sensors transmit measured data over the BLE to the gateway, which then communicate with the upper layer for storage and further processing. The system also includes a clinical governance system that brings both the clinicians and patients in a common platform. It reminds the patient about a scheduled measurement set by the clinicians, notifies the clinicians about any anomalies in the measured data.

Commercial Solutions for Remote Elderly Care

Several remote elderly care solutions are currently available in the market. GreatCall Responder is a small, GPS-enabled device that can easily be attached to a keychain, purse or backpack. It provides an easy and convenient way to safeguard an elderly at home and on-the-go. The user can communicate with a trained service agent by pressing a button on the responder. The agent then assesses the situation and takes further necessary actions. The system also allows the user to contact the EMS directly. MobileHelp uses a GPS-enabled wearable system and offers similar services as GreatCall offers. GrandCare provides in-home healthcare and caregiver services for their clients. The system communicates with the wireless sensors installed in the residence over the internet. Caregivers can log into the GrandCare website to check the health status of the residents. The caregivers are notified if any unusual activities are detected. They also offer a wide range of services including communication and entertainment services to their clients. BeClose remote monitoring system, which is currently owned by Alarm.com, is designed to keep elderly in close contact with their family and caregivers. The system uses discrete wireless sensors placed at different locations in the home to track the daily activities of the elderly. The caregivers or family members of the elderly can also monitor his/her activities using a private and secure webpage. The system can notify the caregivers by phone calls, e-mails or text messages in case of any emergency.

CareSmart Seniors Consulting Inc. (Kelowna, BC, Canada) offers remote monitoring services for the elderly by using a wireless monitoring system from Care Link Advantage. The system utilizes cameras to track the activities of the elderly residing at home or to determine the level of urgency. They consult with the elderly and his/her family to identify the areas of concern and program the system for generating notifications accordingly. In the case of an issue, notifications are sent to the family members and the caregivers via e-mails, text messages and voice messages. Independa offers cloud-based elderly care services through a software platform that uses a smart TV to connect the elderly with the caregivers or the family members. The resident uses a traditional remote controller to switch between TV shows and one of the Independa services. It offers communication services such as video chat, photo sharing, message and alert call between the elderly and the family members. It also reminds key events such as important activities of daily living (ADL), appointments with doctors, social engagements, and schedule of medication.

Currently, many leading communications and media companies such as Rogers Communications, Bell Canada, AT&T and British Telecom (BT) are offering smart home solutions to their customers. Although these solutions offer excellent services for monitoring the safety and security and controlling the environment and the appliances of the home, they still lack comprehensive healthcare monitoring services. Some technology companies such as Philips, ABB and Iqarus are offering remote healthcare services and medical solutions. However, these solutions are primarily designed for large-scale clinical environments.

Samsung, one of the pioneer technology companies, has been working to create a unified platform for elderly care solutions. The platform is designed to be interoperable between Samsung and other devices. With the aid of this unified platform, they are expecting to provide personalized, simple and easy-to-use healthcare solutions, thus offering better care, independence and improved life style for the seniors. Along with ensuring regular communication between the elderly, family members and the healthcare staffs they will also offer seamless connectivity between SMART TVs and appliances, medical alert services, measurement and monitoring of home environment, physiological signs and activities of the seniors.

Research Challenges for Smart Homes

Smart homes allow continuous monitoring of health and activities of the elderly at home as well as monitoring of the environment, safety and security of the home. Although researchers have been working towards a fully functional smart home, there are some challenges that need further research and development in order to improve the overall performance and increase the market penetration of the smart home systems.

First, one of the most pressing concerns for the smart home technologies is associated with the privacy and security of the transmitted data. The data may contain sensitive, protected or confidential information that can endanger residents' privacy and safety, if breached. Therefore, ensuring strong data encryption, database security as well as secured communication channels is critical for smart homes.

Second, smart homes use a wide range of sensors, actuators and other wireless devices, thus generating a large volume of data. Therefore, the communication protocols, hardware and computation resources for the central node of the body area network and wireless sensor network could impose bottlenecks for the seamless and delay-less connectivity as well as data handling capability. The gateway node in wireless sensor network performs extensive data processing as well as communicates with all the components of the system along with the remote server. Robust and efficient algorithms along with effective data compression techniques are the key to optimize the performance of the smart home system.

Third, smart home is a complex system with many discrete devices and systems connected in a common platform. However, the system needs to be carefully designed to deal with integration issues among different devices and also to have optimum number of sensors in order to avoid redundant data, minimize infrastructure and maintenance cost as well as energy consumption without losing key information.

Fourth, the sensing systems of the smart homes, particularly the portable and wearable physiological parameter measurement systems, are aimed for long-term monitoring purposes. Therefore, these systems need to be energy efficient, which can be achieved by using low-power components and efficient batteries. Researchers may also exploit energy harvesting techniques to fulfill the energy requirements of the devices.

Fifth, modularity, expansion capability of the system and interoperability among different smart home platforms are vital for achieving flexibility and widespread acceptance among the users. A modular and extensible structure will allow the users to choose the components from different manufacturers or add/remove services. A common or inter-operable platform for all types of sensors and systems in smart homes is necessary to achieve modularity as well as to ensure flawless and seamless operation. Although, there exists **several hardware-based and IT-based standards at present, they must be converged towards a global common standard** to unfold the full potential of the IoT in smart home and to lay a level playing field for the business competitors as well as the customers.

Sixth, the adoption of AI technologies in the computational platform of the smart home would potentially play a pivotal role in realizing a fully automated and self-sustainable solution. AI technologies, through continuous learning and assessment of the occupants' physiological and behavioral patterns as well as the home environment, will allow the smart homes to make prediction, recommendation and decision about the health, safety and security of the occupants. However, ensuring a highly reliable, accurate and robust implementation of AI technologies particularly for decision making and execution purposes is critical for a trustworthy and safe operation of the smart homes. In addition, in order to make the best use of AI driven features such as machine learning, robotics and big-data computing in the smart home, standardized protocols need to be developed and implemented.

Finally, although many researchers have been working towards smart homes, they mostly addressed some specific aspects of smart homes. A fully functional and comprehensive smart home that addresses all aspects such as home automation, monitoring of residents' health, safety and security, and home environment is still to be realized.

Future Perspectives and Conclusions

In this paper, we have presented a review on the state-of-the-art technologies for elderly care in smart home platforms. The primary objective of the smart homes is to allow the elderly to receive continuous, non-invasive and seamless healthcare service while staying in their convenient home environment. It allows the elderly to minimize their frequency of visits to, or length of stay in expensive healthcare centers such as clinics, hospital and long term care centers, thereby allowing them to lead independent and active lives. Smart homes can also monitor and control the home environment by assessing the behavioral and daily living patterns of the users. The significant advancement in the technology that enables the development of low-power, small and low-cost sensors, and actuators coupled with modern communication technologies paved the way towards realizing continuous monitoring services in a smart home platform from a distant facility.

Smart homes can provide comprehensive information about the overall health status of the elderly through continuous monitoring. Modern low-cost sensors, actuators, computing and communication technologies are the key for developing fully functional smart homes. The system may also include predictive algorithms in future, which will allow it to make predictive decisions about diseases at their early onset by analyzing the monitored data. If a potential health problem is predicted, the system can notify the corresponding healthcare personnel immediately over a secured communication channel for a detailed investigation. This may enable the individual to receive early diagnosis and prevent treatment delay. Researchers may exploit data fusion techniques, which integrate data/information from different sources to develop a predictive tool with a high degree of prediction confidence. The data/information fusion techniques may also allow the system for context-based learning of the residents' daily living and health trends in the smart home.

A key concern for the seamless operation of the smart home system is associated with its energy requirement. Low power consumption and high energy efficiency are critical for the smart home, especially for the wearable and mobile systems used for long-term monitoring purposes. Advanced battery technologies as well as low-power electronic components can be used to increase the operating-time of the system. Researchers also may put their efforts into developing and integrating efficient energy harvesting technologies to fulfill the energy requirements of wearable and mobile systems in the smart home.

Most of the standalone products which are currently available in the market are proprietary and generally developed for one or a few specific tasks or functionalities. Although these systems use standard communication protocols, they are mostly not compatible to, or interoperable with similar systems from other manufacturers, thus leaving the consumers with few alternatives. A common platform for all systems will raise the competition among the manufactures that will result in many alternatives for the consumers, thus increasing the market penetration of smart homes. Therefore, a global industry standard based on a well-defined layered architecture is critical for the widespread acceptance of the smart home technology. Researchers and industry groups may work together to develop and adopt a common and unified industry standard for the smart home system.

Furthermore, as the smart textile technologies continue to evolve, wearable healthcare systems based-on smart textiles are expected to be an attractive solution for comfortable and un-obtrusive monitoring of health parameters in a smart home platform. Textile-based sensors or smart textiles can be fabricated using conventional textile technologies such as weaving, printing, knitting, and stitching, thus having a great potential for developing low-cost wearable sensors. However, further research and development is required to improve the sensitivity, durability, stability, signal-to-noise ratio and reproducibility of the textile-based sensors for using them in long-term monitoring systems.

In recent times, with the development of high performance miniaturized sensors, actuators, computing processors there is a growing interest in implementing innovative and futuristic technologies such as robotics, artificial intelligence (AI) and 3D printing in the healthcare sector. A caring robot driven by AI can assist the elderly in their daily living without any intervention from a third-party system and potentially be a very useful addition to the smart home.

Big communication and media companies, who already have high market penetration and robust infrastructures for high speed and secured data communication, may collaborate with third-party healthcare service providers such as hospitals, clinics, and ambulance services to bring healthcare facilities to the doorsteps of the people. An addition of comprehensive health monitoring systems and healthcare services to their existing smart home solutions can potentially be a giant leap towards a ubiquitous and fully-functional smart home. In fact, some major technology companies such as Samsung, Alarm, and ADT (founded as American District Telegraph) have acquired several small smart home companies in recent years to facilitate health monitoring along with their existing home-security applications in the smart home platform. Also, the industry is still actively working to realize a fully functional smart home-based remote healthcare solution.

Finally, manufacturers also need to pay attention to the design aesthetics in addition to the performance and ease-of-use of the installed devices and systems. A home reflects an individual's personal identity and also creates a sphere of physical and mental comfort for the occupants. Therefore, a superior system with poor visual aesthetics may not be well accepted by the consumers. The architects may also make use of the false walls, interior ceiling, and false ceiling while designing the interior of the home to hide and protect the installed devices and systems, thus providing the occupants with a sense of visual comfort.

Overall, a smart home is a complete system that is expected to bring healthcare, safety and well-being services to the user's doorstep with the aid of modern technologies such as environmental and medical sensors, actuators, high performance computing processors, and wireless commination platforms. The system exploits the concept of Internet-of-Things and connects all sensors and systems of the home to facilitate remote surveillance of the occupants' health as well as the environment, safety and security of the home. Although several standalone systems such as vital sign monitoring, emergency call and reminding systems are available, a fully-fledged smart home is still far from the reality. Therefore, more research and development is required in this sector to develop a fully-functional smart home while ensuring system reliability, privacy and data security, robustness of processing and prediction algorithms, seamless connectivity with minimal transmission delay, energy-efficiency and low setup and maintenance cost.

Wearable Sensors for Health Monitoring

Excerpts from the article "Wearable Sensors for Remote Health Monitoring"
https://www.mdpi.com/1424-8220/17/1/130
Published online by MDPI on **January 2017**.

Remote healthcare monitoring allows people to continue to stay at home rather than in expensive healthcare facilities such as hospitals or nursing homes. It thus provides an efficient and cost-effective alternative to on-site clinical monitoring. Such systems equipped with non-invasive and unobtrusive wearable sensors can be viable diagnostic tools to the healthcare personnel for monitoring important physiological signs and activities of the patients in real-time, from a distant facility.

Wearable devices can monitor and record real-time information about one's physiological condition and motion activities. Wearable sensor-based health monitoring systems may comprise different types of flexible sensors that can be integrated into textile fiber, clothes, and elastic bands or directly attached to the human body.

Listing of some commercial products for monitoring physiological signs and activities.

Product Name	Monitored Parameters	Wireless Platform	Battery Type	Life
Hexoskin® Biometric® Shirt	Heart rate (HR), HR variability, respiratory rate, number of steps, distance traveled, pace, maximal oxygen consumption, and calories burned.	Bluetooth	6–7 days (standalone) 14+ h (multi-training)	
Jawbone UP3™ Fitness Tracker	Sleep stages (REM, light and deep), HR, food and liquid intake, number of steps, distance traveled, running.	Bluetooth LE	Li-ion poly	7 days
Striiv® Fusion Bio Fitness Tracker	HR, number of steps, distance traveled, calories burned, and sleep quality.	Bluetooth LE	Li-ion	5 days
Microsoft® Band 2	HR, calories burned, sleep quality, food, and liquid intake, number of steps, elevation, climbing, running, biking.	Bluetooth	Li-poly	2 days
Fitbit Charge HR™ Fitness Tracker	HR, calories burned, sleep quality, food, and liquid intake, number of steps, elevation, climbing, running.	Bluetooth LE	Li-poly	5–7 days
Garmin vivosmart® HR Fitness Tracker	HR, calories burned, sleep quality, number of steps, climbing, running, swimming.	Bluetooth LE, ANT+	Li-ion	5 days

The sensors are capable of measuring physiological signs such as electrocardiogram (ECG), electromyogram (EMG), heart rate (HR), body temperature, electrodermal activity (EDA), arterial oxygen saturation (SpO2), blood pressure (BP) and respiration rate (RR). In addition, micro-electro-mechanical system (MEMS) based miniature motion sensors such as accelerometers, gyroscopes, and magnetic field sensors are widely used for measuring activity related signals.

Continuous monitoring of physiological signals could help to detect and diagnose several cardiovascular, neurological and pulmonary diseases at their early onset. Also, real-time monitoring of an individual's motion activities could be useful in fall detection, gait pattern and posture analysis, or in sleep assessment.

The wearable health monitoring systems are usually equipped with a variety of electronic and MEMS sensors, actuators, wireless communication modules and signal processing units. The measurements obtained by the sensors connected in a wireless Body Sensor Network (BSN) are transmitted to a nearby processing node using a suitable communication protocol.

The processing node, which could be a Personal Digital Assistant (PDA), smartphone, computer or a custom made processing module based on a microcontroller or a Field Programmable Gate Array (FPGA) runs advanced processing, analysis, and decision algorithms and may also store and display the results to the user. It transmits the measured data over the internet to the healthcare personnel, thus functioning as the gateway to remote healthcare facilities. The general overview of the remote health monitoring system is presented in Figure 1, although actual implemented system could differ depending on the application requirements. For example, some systems can be designed with few numbers of sensors where each of them can send data directly to the nearby gateway. In other systems, the sensors can be connected through a body sensor network (BSN) and the central BSN node gathers data from the sensors, performs limited processing before transmitting the data to the advanced processing platform.

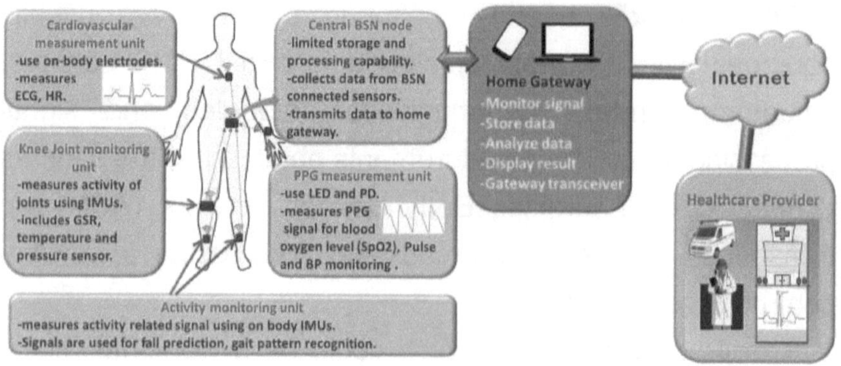

In order to be used for long-term monitoring purposes, wearable health monitoring systems need to satisfy certain medical and ergonomic requirements. For example, the system needs to be comfortable; the components should be flexible, small in dimensions and must be chemically inert, and nontoxic, hypo-allergenic to the human body. In addition, limitation of hardware resources is a major concern for a multi-sensor BSN system where the central node needs to handle a large amount of data coming from different sensor nodes. It also causes significant impact on the system power requirements that needs to be minimized in order to extend the battery life for long-term use.

The measured and processed physiological data are, eventually, transmitted to the remote healthcare facility over the internet. Therefore, it is also necessary to use a secured communication channel in order to safeguard the privacy of sensitive personal medical data.

Cardiovascular Monitoring System

Electrocardiograms (ECGs) represent a non-invasive approach for measuring and recording the fluctuations of cardiac potential.

Only a few numbers of electrodes are used in ambulatory ECG monitoring system at the cost of limited information (Figure c). A continuous ambulatory monitoring device requires a wearable and portable system that could be used comfortably without affecting an individual's daily activities.

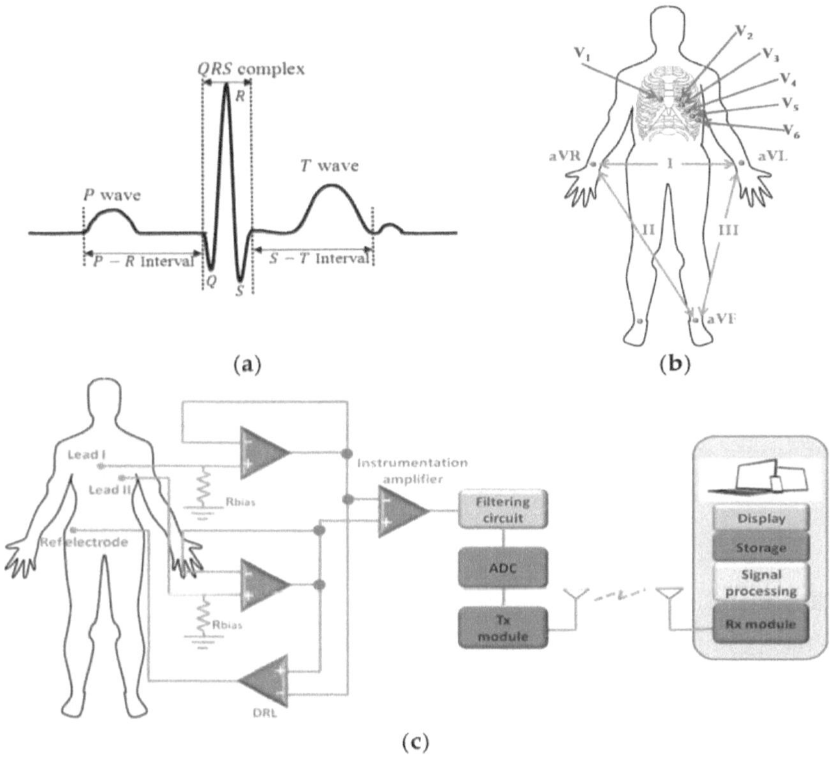

Activity Monitoring System

Monitoring an individual's physical activities and locomotion can be useful in rehabilitation, sports, early detection of musculoskeletal or cognitive diseases, fall and balance assessment. It has been reported that an individual's walking patterns are strongly associated with their health condition.

Abnormality in walking patterns can be indicative of possible musculoskeletal, central nervous system (CNS) or peripheral nervous system diseases.

The walking patterns of ailing people tend to differ from that of normal healthy people. For example, people at the early onset of neurodegenerative disorders such as Alzheimer's or Parkinson's tend to exhibit different walking patterns.

Quantitative analysis and assessment of the gait can be useful for early detection of several diseases, fall prediction as well as during the rehabilitation period after an injury.

Home-based fixed position monitoring, for example, camera-based systems are useful tool for activity monitoring. These systems are capable of recognizing complex gait activities. However, such systems restrict the movement of the user within a specific range. Apart from that, these systems are complex and expensive. In recent years, use of wearable motion sensors such as accelerometers, gyroscopes, and magnetometers are gaining in popularity for measuring human gait activities in real time. The sensors measure linear and angular motion of the body from which a number of key features are extracted.

A schematic of the activity monitoring system based on accelerometers and gyroscopes is presented below.

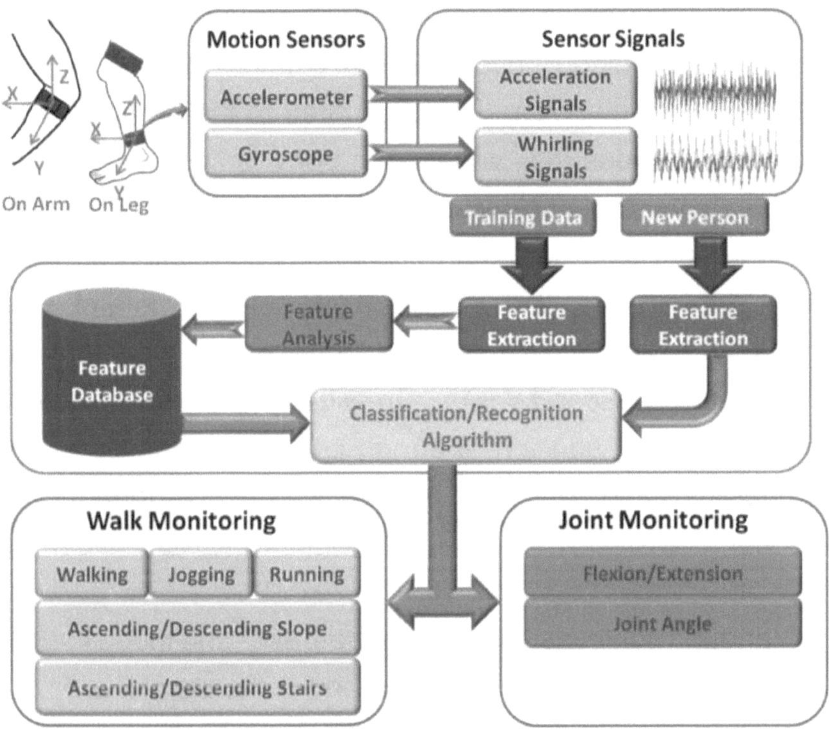

Body Temperature Monitoring System

Body temperature is one of the vital signs that can reflect health conditions. Body temperature increases in infections, malignancy and many inflammatory conditions. Only serial temperature measurements over a long period of time rather than spot checks may prompt the diagnosis. It was reported that core body temperature (CBT) has strong influence on different physiologic conditions as well. Disruptions in the body temperature rhythm are reported to be associated with different types of insomnia. For example, patients suffering from delayed sleep phase insomnia have ~2 h of delay in reaching their minimum CBT compared to the group of good sleepers. Besides this, variation in body temperature rhythm with menstruation cycle was also observed in some studies. Researchers also reported observing a correlation between body temperature and initial stroke severity, infarct size, mortality among stroke patients. It was observed that the infarct size worsens by ~15 mm with 1 °C increase in body temperature. In addition, a strong correlation between body temperature and cognitive functions was also reported in the literature.

Various noninvasive approaches for continuous body temperature monitoring were reported in the literature.

Galvanic Skin Response (GSR) Monitoring System

The autonomic nervous system (ANS) controls and regulates the response of the body to internal or external stimuli by balancing the activities within its two subdivisions: sympathetic and parasympathetic nervous systems. The parasympathetic system, which is also termed as "rest and digest" system conserves and restores energy of the body. On the other hand, the sympathetic system triggers what is often referred to as fight or flight response by increasing metabolic output to deal with the external stimuli. Increased activity of the sympathetic system accelerates heart rate, increases blood pressure, and sweat secretion, as well as prepares the body for motor action by pumping more blood to muscles, lungs, and brain.

Although currently, this information is of no significant clinical use, there is growing interest in many conditions.

A schematic diagram of a wearable GSR monitoring system is presented below.

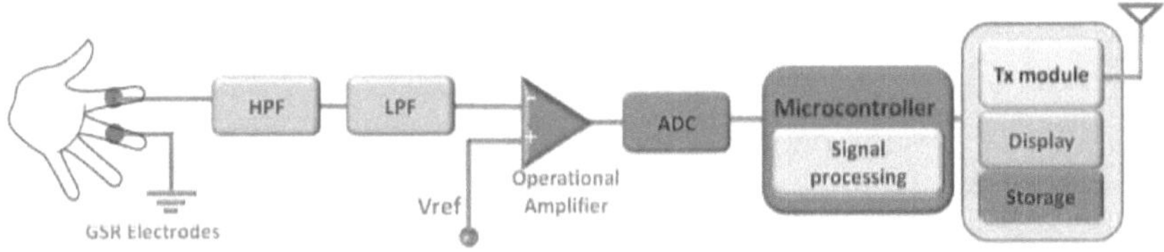

Blood Oxygen Saturation (SpO2) Monitoring Systems

Peripheral capillary oxygen saturation (SpO2) is a measure of the amount of oxygenated hemoglobin in the blood. The oxygen level in blood can be decreased due to health conditions such as cardiovascular diseases, pulmonary diseases, anemia and sleep apnea. It can also be reduced following excessive physical activities. It is essential to maintain an adequate amount of oxygen (>94%) in the blood to ensure proper functioning of cells and tissues. Therefore, it is important to monitor SpO2 continuously, especially for persons having respiratory and heart-related diseases.

Pulse oximeters are widely used as a fast, non-invasive mean to measure the oxygen level in blood. The pulse oximeter usually utilizes red and infrared light emitting diodes (LED) as the light sources. The residue lights after absorption are detected by the photodetector (PD). PPG or SpO2 sensors can be classified into two categories based on the working principles: transmittance and reflectance oximetry (Figure a).

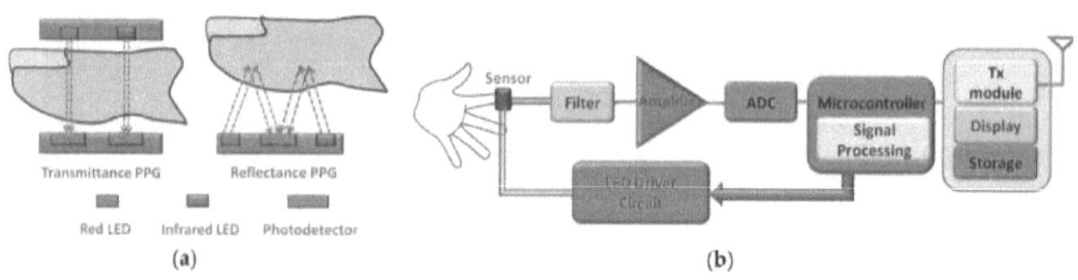

Multi-Sensor Monitoring System

As discussed above, most of the systems were developed aiming to measure or monitor only a specific bio-signal or parameter, for example, only ECG and HR. However, it is necessary to monitor a set of physiological signs such as HR or pulse, BP, respiratory rate, and body temperature; often referred together as vital signs as well as oxygen saturation level in blood and GSR level in order to perform a better assessment of an individual's health condition. Using parameter specific monitoring systems for each parameter is neither practical nor ergonomically sound for continuous and ambulatory monitoring. A network of multiple on-body sensors embedded in a wearable platform along with an on-body data acquisition and transceiver module can be a viable solution for multi-parameter monitoring.

A set of important physiological parameters can be measured and monitored by using four sensors: ECG, PPG, GSR, and temperature sensor.

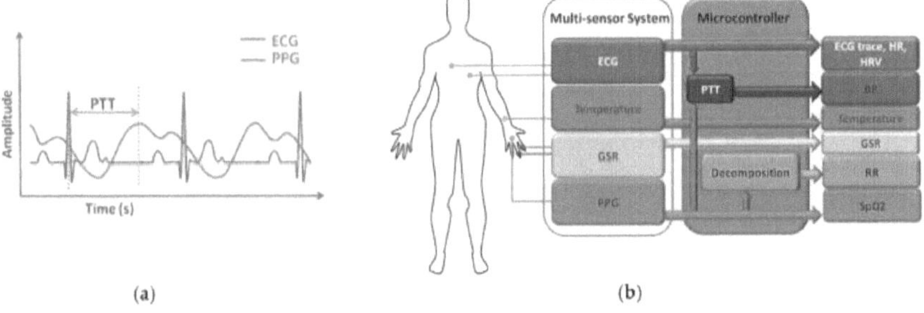

(a)   (b)

Textile-Based Wearable Sensors

Smart textiles associated with healthcare include sensors, actuators, communication, computing, and electronic systems that are made of textile or are suitable for embedding into textiles thus enabling unobtrusive and comfortable means of monitoring physiological signals of the individuals. It makes use of conventional fabric manufacturing techniques such as weaving, knitting, embroidery, and stitching to realize or integrate sensing materials in clothes. Advanced fabrication methods, for example, inkjet-printing, coating, lithography, chemical vapor deposition (CVD) are also used in order to achieve high performance in terms of noise and sensitivity.

Smart textiles can be used to develop wearable on-body electrodes in order to measure electro-physiological signals such as ECG, electroencephalography (EEG), GSR, and electromyography (EMG).

Also, some researchers have used MEMS based inertial sensors such as accelerometers, gyroscopes or magnetic field sensors or their combinations in order to measure the signal corresponding to human locomotion.

Smartphone Sensors for Health Monitoring

Excerpts from the article "Smartphone Sensors for Health Monitoring and Diagnosis"
https://www.mdpi.com/1424-8220/19/9/2164/htm
Published online by MDPI on **May 2019**.

Modern day smartphones come with a number of embedded sensors such as a high-resolution complementary metal-oxide semiconductor (CMOS) image sensor, global positioning system (GPS) sensor, accelerometer, gyroscope, magnetometer, ambient light sensor and microphone. These sensors can be used to measure several health parameters such as heart rate (HR), HR variability (HRV), respiratory rate (RR), and health conditions such as skin diseases and eye diseases, thus turning the communication device into a continuous and long-term health monitoring system.

Table 1 presents the health parameters and conditions that can be monitored using current embedded sensors of the smartphone. The data that are measured by the sensors can be analyzed and displayed on the phone and/or transmitted to a distant healthcare facility or healthcare personnel for further investigation. These existing platforms offer high-speed and seamless internet connectivity even on the go, thereby allowing people to remain connected with their healthcare providers.

Smartphone sensors used for health monitoring.

Monitored Health Issues	Typically Used Smartphone Sensors
Cardiovascular activity e.g., heart rate (HR) and HR variability (HRV)	Image sensor (camera), microphone
Eye health	Image sensor (camera)
Respiratory and lung health	Image sensor (camera), microphone
Skin health	Image sensor camera)
Daily activity and fall	Motion sensors (accelerometer, gyroscope, proximity sensor), Global positioning system (GPS)
Sleep	Motion sensors (accelerometer, gyroscope)
Ear health	Microphone
Cognitive function and mental health	Motion sensors (accelerometer, gyroscope), camera, light sensor, GPS

Table 1 - Smartphone sensors used for health monitoring

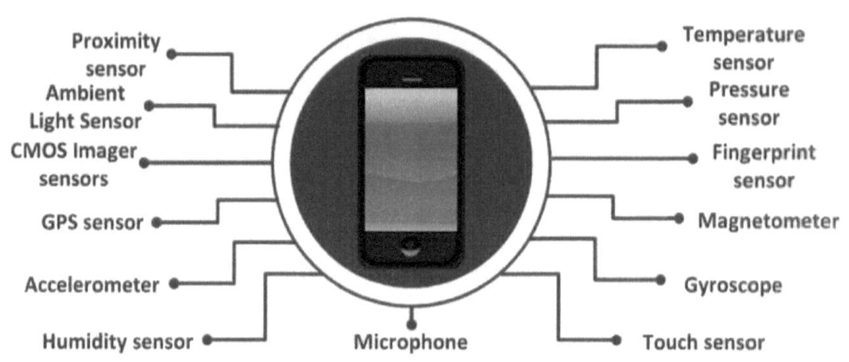

Built-in sensors in a typical present-day smartphone

Smartphones may play a role in enabling a low-cost solution for early diagnosis of diseases such as melanoma, and diabetic retinopathy and remote monitoring of the progression of some diseases.

Bringing Telemedicine into the Home

As the use of telemedicine technologies proliferates, especially among seniors, many of whom have no computer skills, there is a need for effective training approaches to promote basic skills. From telemedicine apps to sensors, today's seniors (and tomorrow's soon-to-be seniors) need to be shown how to live their golden years in their own homes.

The installation of hardware and the training of patients has in the past been done by nurses, usually RNs, of the telemedicine provider.

Technology has long been used to help seniors engage in everyday activities - from user-friendly tablets, laptops and remote control devices (often with larger buttons and quick links to favorite websites and communication tools) to PERS (Personal Emergency Response Service) - the "I've fallen and I can't get up" pendant or wristband.

Telemedicine entrepreneurs and healthcare systems have recognized that health and wellbeing play an increasingly important role in the daily work of seniors and have begun to develop platforms that integrate senior services with healthcare.

With the advent of telemedicine sensors, wearables, PERS pendants, clothing and accessories (such as belts and shoes) have been turned into medical monitors that help seniors monitor their vital signs and daily activities and send this information to the care team.

Some of the more senior-friendly telemedicine technologies include:

Personal Home Assistants - Smart devices like Amazon Alexa and Google Home are used by seniors to remind them of their daily plans, such as: For example, when to take medication, exercise, or take blood pressure or blood glucose readings. They can also summon help (the equivalent of the PERS device at home) or answer simple questions about health and wellbeing.

Intelligent Medicine Containers - Smart pill dispensers and similar telemedicine devices for the home to remind the senior when to take prescriptions, what medications to take, and how much. Some of these devices alert the senior by flashing lights or giving off a particular sound, or they can call out or send a message to the senior's smartphone or tablet. They also measure compliance, record when and how many medications are taken, and sometimes use videos to make sure the senior is taking the drug.

Sensors Embedded in Clothing - Clothes, belts, socks and shoes are being embedded with sensors to measure how a senior moves around, often with the goal of detecting an unsteady gait, evidence of a loss of balance and preventing falls, or alerting the care team when a fall happens. Other garments are equipped with sensors to detect changes in body temperature, heart rate and even irregular movements that may indicate confusion.

The Smart Home (refer to the article above "Smart Homes for Elderly Healthcare") – Thanks to the Internet of Things, a senior's apartment or home can feature a wide variety of telemedicine helpers. These include motion detectors that can track the activity of a senior citizen in the home, including trips to the outdoors, visits to the bathroom, and meals (based on open refrigerator doors, use of the oven or microwave, etc.) connected weight scales; sensor-embedded mattresses that measure sleep and even some vital signs; televisions that include online links to the care team; even personal robots that manage medications, deliver reminders and provide companionship.

While the amount of innovation shows no signs of slowing down, experts expect the connected care platforms of the future to become more intuitive. Home-based platforms will not only relay data back to caregivers, but put that data into the medical record.

Artificial intelligence software will analyze that data and predict a senior's health emergency or fall before it occurs. And a senior released from the hospital will come home to find personalized health and wellness tips, prescription instructions and post-discharge care plans loaded onto the smart TV and/or Tablet.

Following find a write up from AMD…

AMD Global Telemedicine article: How health care practitioners are bringing telehealth into the home

https://www.amdtelemedicine.com/blog/article/how-health-care-practitioners-are-bringing-telehealth-home

In early May, 2018, Regence released promising data for those promoting the value savings of telehealth services. Regence is one of the larger health care payers of the American Midwest and west coast, servicing Idaho, Utah, Oregon and certain counties in Washington State. The company found that consumers are saving $100 on average when they opt for a telehealth appointment rather than an in-person facility visit. This claim factored in the reduced cost of mileage, medical claims and wait times.

These numbers are not surprising, given how much telehealth services have surged in recent years. A report from Foley & Lardner forecasted the overall telehealth industry would grow at a 14.3 percent compound annual growth rate between 2016 and 2020. A data survey conducted by Jackson Healthcare believed that telehealth services would attract seven million active patients by the end of 2018.

Thanks to the technology

Thanks to multiple breakthroughs in technology, telehealth services are more robust than they've ever been. Video streaming allows physicians and other health care officials to speak with and see patients clearly, even over vast distances. This has been especially beneficial for patients in rural and remote areas where a drive to the doctor could take upwards of an hour.

Telehealth services also owe their rapid adoption rate to more accessible greater bandwidth connections. As internet speeds have grown more consistent, real-time medical assistance has become possible. According to Brodie Dychinco, Regence's general manager of convenient care delivery:

"Technology has accelerated the adoption of telehealth as one of many convenient options people have to help contain their health care costs and seek care based on where, when and how they want it."

How exactly are physicians using telehealth services?
There are multiple telehealth software and hardware solutions in existence today. The best software platforms strive to be all-in-one solutions for the patient, that way they don't need to install multiple apps just to cover basic needs.

A robust telehealth platform can allow patients to schedule consultants or simply chat with the next available doctor through secure video or audio. Consumers can also have prescriptions sent to their preferred pharmacy, manage bills and schedule alerts, all from a patient portal that is intuitively accessible.

End of AMD article.

Telemedicine will only benefit seniors if they know it's available

Telemedicine is touted as an important avenue for seniors looking to stay healthy and at home, yet almost 90 percent of seniors recently surveyed said they either don't have access to telemedicine through their Medicare plan or they don't know if they have it.

The survey, conducted by HealthMine, underscores the challenges faced by seniors in connecting to the latest in telemedicine technology: Namely, there hasn't been much effort to get them onto the platform.

Related Articles:

Training Digital Divide Seniors to use a Telehealth System: A Remote Training Approach
https://www.ncbi.nlm.nih.gov/pmc/articles/PMC1839396/

Home Care Providers Find Success Using Telehealth to Connect to Doctors
https://mhealthintelligence.com/news/home-care-providers-find-success-using-telehealth-to-connect-to-doctors

Getting Started in Telehealth
https://www.aap.org/en-us/professional-resources/practice-transformation/telehealth/Pages/Getting-Started-in-Telehealth.aspx

Home Medical Exam Kit (Edition II)

Get a complete medical exam wherever you are with TytoCare TytoHome. This electronic health care device allows you to receive on-demand physical exams via live video chat with a doctor's office using an exam camera and a basal thermometer and otoscope, stethoscope and tongue depressor adapters. This HIPAA-secure TytoCare TytoHome digital device transmits test results to an electronic health record for easy monitoring.

TytoCare TytoHome Medical Exam Kit White G 1.5 - Best Buy

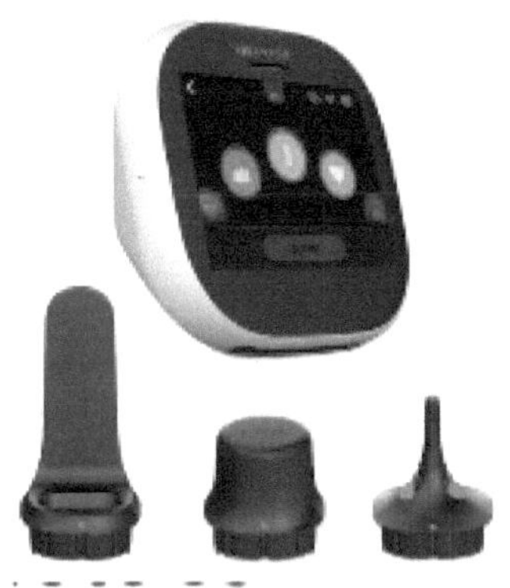

Connect with a doctor 24/7

Download the free TytoApp™ for most iOS and Android devices to get a video consult from a licensed medical provider. Tyto goes beyond a phone or video chat with a doctor by providing an on-demand, clinic-quality medical exam right from your home.

Use the included instruments

From an otoscope (ears) and stethoscope (heart, lungs, and abdomen) to a basal thermometer and digital camera (skin and throat), Tyto is designed to provide your doctor with the same type of data they would use in the office.

Conduct your own exam

Tyto's proprietary guidance technology ensures that anyone can capture and share accurate results.

Get a diagnosis

The physician will use the data provided by Tyto and the video consult to examine, diagnose, and treat your conditions remotely. This can include a treatment plan and a prescription sent directly to your pharmacy if needed.

Treat common conditions

Including ear infections, sore throats, fever, cold and flu, allergies, pink eye, nausea, constipation, asthma, bronchitis, upper respiratory infections, bug bites and common skin conditions, including contact dermatitis, rash and diaper rash.

Keep your information secure

Tyto uses a HIPAA-secure platform that only you and the doctor can access, so you can be certain your information is safe and secure. And all TytoCare products are FDA-cleared and comply with FDA standards.

Talk to trusted physicians

Tyto works with qualified and experienced physicians around the country. Each doctor goes through a rigorous selection process to become a part of the network.

Use Tyto anywhere

Tyto is lightweight, compact, and portable so you can use it anywhere. All you need is the TytoApp, a smartphone or tablet, and a Wi-Fi connection. It is recommended that adults aged 18-65 operate the device.

Pay $60 or less per medical exam

You can use your health insurance or HSA/FSA account up front – or ask your provider or insurance company if they offer reimbursements for virtual medical exams or telehealth visits.

The health provider network will be set according to the geolocation of the device and is subject to change. Exam prices will vary depending on your health provider, your insurance or HSA/FSA provider. Reimbursements may not apply. Subject to insurance and provider term & conditions.

Product Name: TytoHome Medical Exam Kit

Model Number: G 1.5

Dimension: 3.35 x 0.1 x 2.87 inches

Product Weight: 0.33 pounds

Accessories Included: Otoscope adapter, Stethoscope adapter, Tongue depressor, USB cord, Rechargeable battery.

FROM THE MANUFACTURER:

Your On-Demand Medical Exam

Tyto is a handheld exam kit and app that lets you perform guided medical exams, with a doctor, anytime, anywhere. With Tyto, you can receive a diagnosis from your doctor, a treatment plan, and a prescription if needed -- all from the comfort of home.

To ER or not to ER?

It's 2 am and your child can't stop crying. Is it serious? Do you need to rush to urgent care, the hospital, or neither? Is it worth risking a germ-infested waiting room if you aren't sure? Tyto helps answer these questions by connecting you directly with your doctor for a live medical exam. Right when you need it. Right from home.

Sick? Or really sick?

Some kids seem to get sick all the time, with ear infections, pink eye, fevers, rashes, cold, cough, or just some good old-fashioned congestion. Tyto enables your doctor to diagnose those common conditions without having to go all the way to the office.

Notice

The above article was printed on the web site of Best Buy. No responsibility is assumed for the accuracy of the content.

Teladoc faces rising Competition (Edition II)

Telemedicine article: Teladoc Will Face Increasing Competition And Pricing Pressure

https://seekingalpha.com/article/4314623-teladoc-will-face-increasing-competition-and-pricing-pressure

Summary

- Virtual healthcare is a logical step to cut costs and improve services in the behemoth that is US healthcare, hence the market has excellent growth prospects.

- That growth has boosted the fortunes of Teladoc Health, the market leader in virtual healthcare.

- While Teladoc's growth, scale and scope is impressive, we think that the virtual healthcare market has low barriers to entry and competition will be increasing.

- We see several types of new entrants and even a potential shift in consumer expectations towards zero-cost provision of virtual care.

Recently, we wrote about the spectacular growth of Teladoc Health (TDOC), the leader in virtual healthcare. The reason for that is actually quite simple: virtual healthcare offers important advantages in cost and convenience.

According to a Fortune Business Insight study:

The global virtual reality in the healthcare market size stood at USD 1.56 Billion in 2018 is expected to reach USD 30.40 Billion by 2026, exhibiting a CAGR of 42.4%

We have little doubt that Teladoc, as the market leader, will be benefiting from a big tailwind like this. However, thinking about the market, we see that the industry has fairly low barriers to entry and see competition from several main sources:

- Other big virtual healthcare providers
- Caregivers going digital
- Companies building their own solutions and potentially opening these up for third parties
- Insurance companies offering virtual care by teaming up with providers

The reality is that both barriers to entry and the cost of virtual care are low, which makes it a very attractive proposition for new types of competition to enter the market.

Caregivers

Doctors and specialists, practices and even entire hospitals can associate, install conference tech and offer virtual healthcare. For instance, take Novant Health, an integrated system of physician practices, hospitals and outpatient centers, started providing online services early in the decade. From The Charlotte Observer:

In 2011, Novant Health debuted its MyChart online portal offering greater patient access to doctors and medical records. Today, MyChart is being used in eight hospitals and more than 400 physician practices in three states. About 400,000 patients have enrolled, and about 200,000 are logging in at least once a month.

Through the website, www.mynovant.org, patients can view their medical history and test results, check immunization records and medicines, schedule appointments, renew prescriptions, send messages and pictures to their doctor's office, and pay bills. These functions are also available through an app for mobile devices. Search under MyChart and select Novant Health.

MyChart is accessible to anyone, even patients without a Novant doctor. On the "Physician Finder" function, patients can choose their own doctor or one they've never met, and click to make an appointment in real time. Novant patients have been using MyChart to schedule video visits and make e-visits with their personal physicians for more than a year... Novant plans to begin offering unscheduled video visits sometime in 2015.

More recently, Novant has been taking it a step further and added some simple diagnostic technology, leveraging virtual healthcare. From WBTV:

Novant Health is expanding access to healthcare using a device called TytoHome. TytoHome is a device that patients can use to communicate with physicians via video chat. Unlike other video visits with a doctor, TytoHome gives doctor's the ability to examine the patient too. "It allows us to do more than just look at a patient, it allows us to examine a patient. For example, look in the ear, throat, listen to the heart, a heart rate, it gives a temperature," Family Physician Dr. Aram Alexanian said. The TytoHome device comes with attachments that a patient can use on themselves. The images captured are viewed in real time by a physician during the video chat. TytoHome comes with a thermometer attachment, stethoscope adaptor, tongue depressor, and otoscope adaptor. The attachments give doctors the ability to view a patient's temperature, heart rate, ears, throat, and listen to a patient's lung and abdominal sounds through video chat.

This isn't all that difficult to do, and we wonder why more providers don't do it, as it seems an obvious thing to do, saving cost and time for everybody involved. The obvious thing to start is video conferencing tech - enter video conferencing technology company Zoom Video Communications (ZM). From the company's blog:

Today Zoom announced that we have developed the industry's first scalable, cloud-based video telehealth service, Zoom for Telehealth, featuring an integration with electronic health record system Epic. Zoom for Telehealth offers a standard feature set for healthcare enterprises and providers, enabling reliable, HIPAA-compliant communications between organizations, care teams, and patients.

Zoom for Telehealth includes the following features pre-configured:

- Cloud-based video, audio, and content sharing
- Support for desktop, mobile, and conference room systems
- Epic integration enabled
- End-to-end AES-256 bit encryption of all meeting data and instant messages
- Signed Business Associate Agreement (BAA) to enable HIPAA compliance
- Waiting room for patient privacy enabled
- Platform API/SDK for integration with healthcare applications to streamline workflows
- Remote camera control enabled
- Integration with point-of-care peripherals

We know that Teladoc is growing big on mental health, which is a natural fit for virtual healthcare, but Zoom is emerging here as well, enabling Regroup, one of the leading telepsychiatry companies in the U.S. From the company blog:

In addition to using Zoom Meetings for sales demos and one-to-one patient engagement, Regroup leverages Zoom Video Webinars to establish thought leadership in its industry by educating hundreds of viewers at a time, as well as creating evergreen content that lives on the company blog after the webinar is over.

"We went from 0 to 75 customers in 23 states, providing services to 170-plus clinical sites, and from 0 to 100,000 virtual meetings a year over Zoom. Most importantly, Zoom enabled people in access-challenged geographies to get mental healthcare that they simply wouldn't be able to get otherwise," Cohn said.

Zoom sees its videoconferencing and additional technologies as a substantial growth market taking its already considerable TAM well beyond that of UCaaS. It has developed a string of solutions for the industry.

Basically, this more or less off-the-shelf technology enables medical facilities to embark on DIY virtual healthcare.

Amazon

Amazon (AMZN) is also moving into healthcare:

- Acquiring online pharmacy PillPack.
- Partnering with healthcare organizations to develop Alexa skills handling patient information.

- Haven Healthcare, the partnership with JPMorgan and Berkshire Hathaway creating a new healthcare insurance company offering various plans to its employees.
- Creating Amazon Care, providing employees with virtual healthcare.

It's Amazon Care that is of immediate interest here, as Amazon has partnered with Oasis Medical Group to provide the virtual healthcare service to its employees in Seattle, and the idea is to expand this to all its employees. From The Verge:

Once an employee signs up, they can either chat with a clinician over text or a video call, getting anything from advice to a diagnosis on the fly. If the nurse or doctor you're chatting with thinks you need a closer assessment they can recommend something called Mobile Care, which will literally send a nurse to your home, office, or other spot in Seattle.

According to the website, "the Mobile Care nurse may collect lab samples, perform some onsite testing (such as strep tests), administer common vaccines, or perform physical examinations."

We can't help but think that while this is intended for Amazon employees, there is no inherent reason, or limitation, to extend it beyond the realm of its own employees, and we're not the only ones (Business Insider):

Back in June, statements from JPMorgan CEO Jamie Dimon seemed to suggest that Haven may have a future beyond supplying health coverage to employees of its three parent companies, even if it may take years to do so. But with so much capital and the JV's combined resources behind it, we believe Haven certainly has the potential to push in and disrupt the $670 billion private insurance market. JPMorgan and Amazon have made major health acquisitions since announcing Haven - and they could be laying the groundwork to disrupt the healthcare industry across the board.

The explicit goal of Haven (a non-profit insurer) is to bring down the cost of healthcare, and it is experimenting with different kinds of policies that offer incentives (like lower co-pays, deductibles, prescription costs, etc.) if members meet various health goals (like blood pressure, weight, etc.).

However, Haven doesn't own healthcare facilities itself. While its sheer size could start to have a moderating effect on prices, it depends on negotiating prices with hospitals and other providers of care.

But virtual care offers an obvious starting point to produce a sizable effect on the cost of care, and this is exactly what Amazon is doing with Amazon Care. From Motley Fool:

A virtual visit is $472 less expensive than an in-office visit, according to Veracity Analytics.

This might not even capture all the savings, as lowering care access barriers is likely to increase preventive care, especially when combined with the kind of incentives that Haven is experimenting with.

The cost savings are so substantial that other health insurers have noticed. Here is one, Oscar Health, that is offering virtual care for free. From The Business Journals (our emphasis):

Oscar Health aims to use technology to make health care more personalized and transparent. For example, **Oscar customers have free telemedicine access 24/7** and have a personalized concierge team to help coordinate care.

"The general gist is that for the past two years, we've been moving more and more away from tele-urgent care and more towards tele-primary care," Schlosser said.

As part of Oscar Health's focus on virtual primary care, Schlosser said the provider soon will let members pick their own "virtual primary care physician" who caters to the patient's personal needs, whether it be a deep knowledge of chronic conditions or a specialty area.

While we're not there yet, and it might not even happen, we hate to think what would happen to Teladoc's business if Amazon would start to offer Haven and Amazon Care to all prime members, with virtual visits at zero cost.

Conclusion

While virtual healthcare offers tremendous growth opportunities for the likes of Teladoc, the barriers to entry are rather low. While Teladoc, as the market leader, is ahead of its direct competition, other competitors are emerging that could make life more difficult for the company.

Technological developments like the advent of 5G and teleconferencing solutions from the likes of Zoom enable smaller players, like hospitals and medical practices, to offer their own virtual healthcare, competing from below.

Then, there are big companies like Amazon that offer virtual care for their employees and could very well open this up to the wider public when they have worked out the details and get the infrastructure in place.

Or insurance companies like Oscar Health, teaming up with provider networks to offer virtual care, at zero cost. The latter especially is a threat to the likes of Teladoc, as it might shift customer expectations like Amazon's free same-day shipping has.

This doesn't mean that there is no market for the likes of Teladoc. Not every big company (let alone smaller ones) can or will start its own virtual healthcare initiative like Amazon. For those that can't, there are ready-made alternatives like Teladoc, and they only have to sign up.

So, while we see no immediate threat to Teladoc's growth, we do see a gradual erosion of its pricing power as virtual care becomes more established, and this is simply a reflection of the low barriers to entry and low marginal cost of virtual care.

Telemedicine focused on Infectious Disease (Edition II)

In consideration of a JAMA Health Forum Viewpoint (published January 23, 2020) on Coronavirus Infections, the following article related to **a new telemedicine company focused on Infectious Disease – ID** - may be of significance.

JAMA Network begins with: Human coronaviruses (HCoVs) have long been considered inconsequential pathogens, causing the "common cold" in otherwise healthy people. However, in the 21st century, 2 highly pathogenic HCoVs - severe acute respiratory syndrome coronavirus (SARS-CoV) and Middle East respiratory syndrome coronavirus (MERS-CoV) - emerged from animal reservoirs to cause global epidemics with alarming morbidity and mortality. In December 2019, yet **another pathogenic HCoV, 2019 novel coronavirus (2019-nCoV), was recognized in Wuhan, China**, and has caused serious illness and death. The ultimate scope and effect of this outbreak is unclear at present as the situation is rapidly evolving.

JAMA concludes: While the trajectory of this outbreak is impossible to predict, effective response requires prompt action from the standpoint of classic public health strategies to the timely development and implementation of effective countermeasures. The emergence of yet another outbreak of human disease caused by a pathogen from a viral family formerly thought to be relatively benign underscores the perpetual challenge of emerging infectious diseases and the importance of sustained preparedness.

Article: UPMC launches new telemedicine company focused on infectious disease – ID Connect

Diagnosis and treatment of disease and antibiotic-resistant bacteria is complex and challenging for small hospitals, who could care for patients with remote help from top-tier infectious disease experts.

https://www.healthcareitnews.com/news/upmc-launches-new-telemedicine-company-focused-infectious-disease

UPMC has launched a new company, Infectious Disease Connect, that seeks to boost ID services using telehealth technology – helping providers improve outcomes and lower costs by reducing transfers and treating patients in their own communities.

WHY IT MATTERS

UPMC already offers infectious disease services to some patients via telemedicine and has for several years. It enables fewer relocations to tertiary care facilities, helps reduce nosocomial infections and decreases misuse of antibiotics, say UPMC officials – who note that such interventions can also result in shorter hospital stays, lower readmissions and reduced mortality rates for hospitals.

Add to this the fact that there is a shortage nationwide of ID specialists, even as the risks, costs regulatory requirements of infectious diseases and healthcare-associated infections are increasing, and the appeal of telemedicine in this area is apparent, especially as hospitals and health systems aim to succeed in value-based care.

ID Connect, launched UPMC Enterprises, the health system's innovation and commercialization arm, was co-founded by Rima Abdel-Massih, MD, director of tele-ID services at UPMC, and John Mellors, MD, chief of the Division of Infectious Diseases at UPMC and the University of Pittsburgh, are co-founders of the new company.

The startup already serves 10 UPMC and five non-UPMC hospitals in the Pennsylvania region. As it rolls out, it will focus first on smaller hospitals with fewer than 300 beds.

"These smaller facilities face an especially difficult time recruiting and retaining already scarce ID specialists," said Abdel-Massih, who will serve as chief medical officer. "ID Connect can cost-effectively provide ID specialists, full-time or part-time, to augment existing staff."

The company will at first be staffed by UPMC-based infectious disease specialists, but as it grows it will be hiring other clinicians for patient consultations, and seeking outside expertise in antimicrobial stewardship and infection prevention and control, according to ID Connect President David Zynn.

THE LARGER TREND

Zynn notes that HAIs affect 5 to 10 percent of patients and can cost hospitals more than $40 million each year. Those cost increases are further exacerbated by unnecessary prescriptions that can cause adverse side effects or contribute to antibiotic resistance. With many hospitals losing ground in the fight against HAIs, any innovative tool to help in the battle is useful.

As we've been showing during our focus on digital transformation, sing telemedicine to help hospitals more efficiently and effectively treat infection could be a boon for the small providers ID Connect is targeting for its initial business.

ON THE RECORD

"As diagnosing and treating infectious diseases and 'superbugs' become increasingly complex, having access to infectious disease experts will be essential for every health care facility," said Zynn. "Created by a health system that has led the way in both managing infectious diseases and implementing telemedicine, ID Connect is well-positioned to effectively serve hospitals and their patients."

"With the growing threat of drug-resistant organisms and costly government penalties for health care-associated infections, it has never been more critical for hospitals to properly diagnose, treat and prevent such infections," said Abdel-Massih. "However, with ID specialists in short supply, many hospitals, especially smaller, community facilities, are struggling to meet this need. ID Connect was created to fill that gap."

Note: The University of Pittsburgh Medical Center (UPMC) is a $20 billion integrated global health enterprise that has 87,000 employees.

Telemedicine: Middle-aged Adults Care

AMD Global Telemedicine article: Telemedicine in Life Stages: Middle-aged adults.

https://www.amdtelemedicine.com/blog/article/telemedicine-life-stages-middle-aged-adults

Over the last decade, technology has completely transformed the way we go about our everyday lives. Since it's all the younger population has ever known, it's easier for adolescents and teens to get on board with digital assets in the world of health care. However, telemedicine is a tool that can benefit anyone down the life cycle, regardless of age, and older adults are becoming more inclined to consider this option. In fact, a survey by The Associated Press-NORC Center for Public Affairs Research found that more than half of Americans over the age of 40 feel comfortable using a video service for a medical consultation, and 88% would feel comfortable using telemedicine to receive care and manage chronic illness.

As a part of the Telemedicine in Life Stages series, we recently covered adolescents and young adults. This edition will dive into the next stage of life in regard to older adults and the role telehealth plays in the care continuum, touching on common conditions that become more prevalent at this age such as concerns with cardiovascular health, obesity and dementia risks.

Cardiovascular health

Elevated blood pressure and cholesterol levels have a major impact on the heart; both are associated with cardiovascular health issues that could lead to heart attack, stroke, heart disease or even death.

Patients with any of these conditions may find themselves in and out of the doctor's office - or even worse, the hospital - when health concerns arise. According to a study by the College of Health Professions at Texas State University, however, telemedicine has the ability to reduce hospitalizations and readmission rates and improve health outcomes and overall patient satisfaction. This is due to the opportunity to monitor outpatient care from remote or rural areas since distance is a common barrier that keeps patients from receiving the assistance they need.

Obesity

The National Institute of Diabetes and Digestive and Kidney Diseases reported that the National Health and Nutrition Examination Survey found more than 1 in 3 adults were considered overweight, while 2 in 3 adults were considered obese. This issue is commonly associated with unhealthy eating and physical inactivity, but may also be due to uncontrollable factors like genes, medical illnesses and medications.

With so many individuals affected by this condition, more people should focus on getting resources to better their overall health. The idea of eating well and exercising more isn't enough; patients need guidance to address the issue of obesity. Telemedicine has the ability to do just this: A recent study published in the Journal of Telemedicine and Telecare found that 69% of patients who followed a 12-week telehealth-based weight loss program saw significant weight loss. One of the main features of the program was health coaching via video conference, which enabled patients to reach out to dietitians and other medical professionals to stay on track. A key element to the success of this type of program is having the flexibility to see patients on demand via a telehealth application where patients can connect with a clinician on the spot or scheduled a future virtual appointment.

Dementia

While dementia is most common in older adults aged 65 and above, it's not just a disease of old age. According to the Alzheimer's Association, around 5% of the 5 million Americans living with Alzheimer's disease have younger onset dementia, affecting hundreds of thousands of adults in their 40s and 50s.

Dementia patients, especially those in the early stages of the disease, can benefit from receiving care via telemedicine. It enables them to go to a nearby clinic and gain immediate access to a specialist who may be too far away to meet face-to-face. This allows dementia patients to receive the care they need without worrying about the barrier of distance, which also alleviates the burden of timely travel on caregivers.

Telemedicine and telehealth technologies remove some of the barriers for adults with chronic conditions and enables them to receive proper and timely care. Leveraging a virtual care model allows healthcare professionals to improve patient engagement, make more informed decisions on patient care and increase the continuity of care. If you're interested in providing a more convenient option for your patient population, reach out to AMD Global Telemedicine.

Related Articles:

Optimizing your telemedicine workflow
https://www.amdtelemedicine.com/blog/article/optimizing-your-telemedicine-workflow

Telemedicine in Life Stages: Elderly care
https://www.amdtelemedicine.com/blog/article/telemedicine-life-stages-elderly-care

Telemedicine: Elderly Care

AMD Global Telemedicine article: Telemedicine in Life Stages: Elderly care.

https://www.amdtelemedicine.com/blog/article/telemedicine-life-stages-elderly-care

When you think about the impact telemedicine has on individuals throughout the life cycle, it's no secret that this technology is revolutionary in this day and age and is becoming more frequently used and respected. From infancy and teen care to aiding older adults, the advantages of telehealth benefit every age group.

As the final staple in our Telemedicine in Life Stages series, this article will dive into the next stage of life, elderly care, and the role telemedicine plays in the care continuum. We'll discuss diseases and conditions that are most commonly faced by elders, as well as the impact telehealth has on transforming the patient care models at long-term care facilities.

Greater access to specialty care

In part 3 of our series, we touched on dementia and the impact early onset has on middle-aged adults. The statistics are more severe for the elderly, however - the Alzheimer's

Association reported that 1 in 10 people aged 65 and older have Alzheimer's.

Telemedicine can be especially beneficial to older adults who need regular assistance. Instead of traveling a great distance to see a specialist, they can head to a nearby clinic to receive complementary care via telehealth. This eliminates the stress that comes with travel and enables seniors to feel more comfortable by seeking care near home.

The same goes for other needs for specialty care. According to the National Council on Aging, about 80% of the elderly population live with at least one chronic condition, 77% reportedly have at least two diseases. Diabetes, arthritis, cataracts, glaucoma and kidney issues are among the common conditions faced by the elderly population. Those who have cases severe enough to seek assistance from a specialist may find it more difficult when there's a travel barrier. Telemedicine enables greater access to specialty care by offering a telehealth conference with a specialist in a nearby clinic.

Telemedicine in long-term care facilities

For some older adults, chronic conditions can become so severe or potentially life-threatening that the need to stay in a long-term care facility arises. With this style of facility comes constant discharge, readmission and new admission, however, which can cause a lack in coordination of care. If there's an issue that cannot be taken care of within the facility, for example, staff members may discharge a patient and send them to a hospital or skilled facility to address the problem - only to readmit said patient after the condition is considered under control again.

Using telemedicine in long-term care facilities improves the model of care and patient outcomes. Instead of sending a patient back to the hospital for a change of condition, nurses and medical staff members can use a telehealth consult to connect with a specialist and address questions or concerns in regard to a disease or condition. This keeps the patient in the facility which reduces readmissions and can improve overall patient satisfaction. Immediate access to care is the most important and beneficial aspect of telemedicine in long-term care settings. When aging adults are in need of specialty care, too long of a wait time can be detrimental to health. Fast response times are necessary, and telemedicine can gain elderly adults quick access to the care they need as soon as possible.

Aging in place

When it comes to growing older, most adults agree that aging in place is the optimal choice. For many, there's comfort in staying in a longtime home over downsizing and living in a nursing facility instead. However, the issue with access to necessary care comes to light when seniors prefer to stay in their homes. Telemedicine has the ability to honor the idea of aging in place - older adults can receive specialty care at a nearby clinic instead of uprooting their entire life from their homes. This reduces the stress that can come with aging and can improve the overall satisfaction of life for older adults.

Telemedicine enables elderly adults to receive the care they need when common barriers get in the way. With a virtual care model, your organization can assist elderly adults in a timely, efficient manner and help them make better-informed decisions towards a healthier and happier way of life. If you're interested in improving patient satisfaction and increasing continuity of care, contact AMD Global Telemedicine today. We have a telehealth solution for you.

Related Articles:

Telemedicine in Life Stages: Middle-aged adults.
https://www.amdtelemedicine.com/blog/article/telemedicine-life-stages-middle-aged-adults

How on-demand telemedicine can assist with allergies
https://www.amdtelemedicine.com/blog/article/how-demand-telemedicine-can-assist-allergies

IT Infrastructure for Telemedicine

As healthcare organizations increase the utilization of telemedicine programs, it is important to ensure that all health IT infrastructure requirements for telemedicine are met. Organizations that fail to properly support their telemedicine network will experience security risks, and dissatisfied clinicians and patients.

Developing a plan that addresses current telemedicine needs as well as future demands is the first thing organizations need to do when planning for telemedicine. The network must be scalable and updates need to be made on a realistic timeline that takes budget and available resources into account.

Telemedicine is an important tool, especially for rural hospitals that treat patients who cannot make frequent trips to their providers. These areas often have weaker connectivity than urban areas, which makes telemedicine infrastructure critical for supporting these areas.

Telemedicine/telehealth programs require:
- <u>Access to broadband internet</u>: Sufficient bandwidth is needed to transmit audio and video data. Organizations in rural areas may have difficulty connecting to or obtaining affordable and reliable broadband service.

- <u>Imaging devices</u>: These devices are the backbone of telemedicine and allow healthcare organizations to see and hear patients even when they are miles apart. Digital stethoscopes, for instance, can transmit heart and lung sounds to remote providers.
- <u>Access to technical support staff</u>: Technical support staff members can help answer telemedicine program questions.
- <u>Staff training</u>: Staff must be trained to use telemedicine technology, which may take time. Organizations should consider whether workflow changes may be required and train accordingly.

Telemedicine is about reliable connectivity no matter where the clinician or patient is located. **Unreliable connectivity will prevent any telemedicine program from being successful.**

Organizations must consider how clinicians and patients are securely connecting to the network remotely. Businesses also need to know how strong that connection is to support video streaming and other data intensive telemedicine needs.

Organizations need to compensate for lack of coverage and set up telemedicine programs that can take advantage of whichever signal is the strongest and most reliable in the region.

This may require organizations to have multiple contracts with different cellular or wireless providers in different areas, which can be especially complex for larger healthcare organizations.

A growing population, more people living with chronic disease, and the desire for people to consult with specialists that are not in their region results in a telemedicine use increase.

IT entities need to start with a realistic plan as the first step in building a network that will support the connectivity and security requirements of the expanding telemedicine data. Once a plan is created, they should reach out to telemedicine vendors and consult with them while planning out infrastructure upgrades that will help organizations establish a solid network without gaps.

Relying on just one Wi-Fi provider is not reliable or secure enough for clinicians to successfully exchange the information they need to treat and communicate with patients. Building a scalable IT infrastructure to support telemedicine is necessary for telemedicine companies.

Businesses also need to consider the new 5G cellular connections for areas that don't have reliable or secure Wi-Fi. **It is predicted that the 5G network might even replace the traditional home Internet connections that run on Wi-Fi.**

Telemedicine tools that can connect to the strongest signal, whether it's Wi-Fi or cellular, can also safeguard the increase of signal quality.

Related Article:

Health IT Infrastructure Supports Successful Telemedicine Programs

https://hitinfrastructure.com/news/health-it-infrastructure-supports-successful-telemedicine-programs

Successful telemedicine programs depend heavily on health IT infrastructure and how the remote patients and clinicians can access the network.

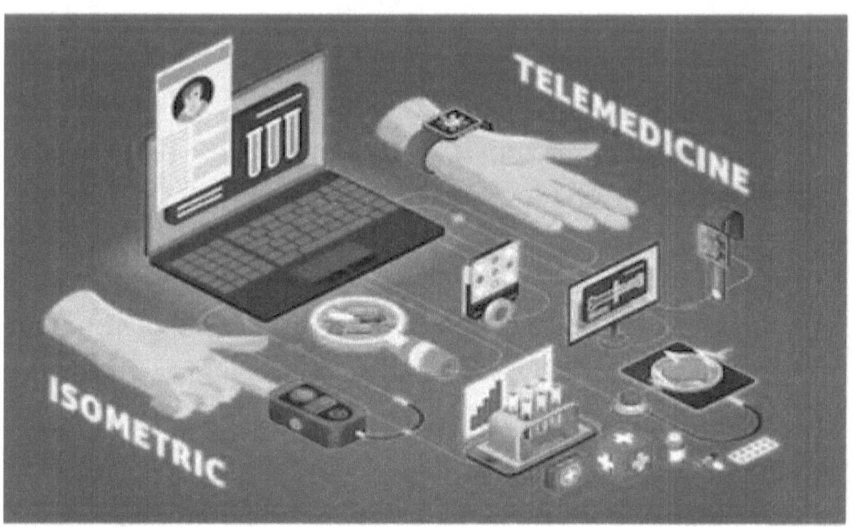

Health IT infrastructure is significantly impacted by the growing popularity of telemedicine, with clinicians and patients able to take advantage of innovative tools.

Patient convenience and cutting back costs are two benefits of telemedicine, but setting up a successful telemedicine program from an infrastructure perspective needs a significant amount of attention.

Using Broadband to Support IoMT

Excerpts of an article from HIT Infrastructure:

Using Broadband to Support Internet of Medical Things

Organizations working with the Internet of Medical Things (IoMT) need to consider broadband to ensure their devices are successfully connecting and communicating with the network.

https://hitinfrastructure.com/features/using-broadband-to-support-internet-of-medical-things

Healthcare organizations are adopting Internet of Medical Things (IoMT) devices to connect patients and clinicians to the network. IoMT devices provide remote monitoring solutions for patients and collect valuable data that can be used for analytics.

These connected healthcare devices save organizations money by keeping patients out of the hospital. Monitoring patients with IoMT devices reduces the rate of return visits and gives clinicians better insight into a patient's conditions.

However, the influx of IoMT devices can put strain on the network infrastructure leading to bottlenecking, which prevents clinicians from accessing vital information when they need it.

Large organizations can have up to three times more connected medical devices than traditional computers and smartphones. These connected IoT devices put massive strain on the network and can cause outages if the traffic is not managed and monitored properly.

The weight of traffic from these devices also makes connecting them via the present IT network impractical. Many healthcare organizations are using broadband to connect IoMT devices used on campus and for remote care.

Broadband is becoming a more attractive and realistic option for healthcare organizations to overcome these IoMT connectivity issues.

Broadband offers more reliable connections and allows device users to be truly mobile. However, organizations need to consider how IoMT devices are built to ensure they can properly connect to the broadband network.

Organizations must also consider what access patients have to broadband and make efforts to ensure rural communities can use broadband for telemedicine programs.

Using Antennas to Connect to Broadband

The success of IoMT devices begins with how they are built. The device's antenna must be properly placed and configured or the device will not work as intended. Medical devices are notoriously noisy and are made up of many different parts that may disrupt the antenna's signal if not properly positioned.

The antenna is the link to network connectivity and converts electrical signal into radio waves, which is why it's critical for IoMT devices to have efficient antennas. A good antenna makes all the difference, especially when it comes to fringe areas or areas with bad signals. This is vital to telemedicine and telehealth programs that provide remote care in rural areas.

While there are many benefits from healthcare IoT devices, organizations often face challenges in the design and testing phases of medical device development because they may lack awareness of the antenna and its necessary certifications.

For example, there's a lot of high powered electronics inside a defibrillator. There are mechanisms in place that create a lot of RF noise and there's nothing you can do to change that. It's the nature of a defibrillator. When you go to cellular or any wireless technology, that becomes very challenging. If the antenna is not efficient, the device is working harder to maintain or get that connectivity. The less efficient the antenna is the more power the device will consume.

Organizations need to communicate with medical device companies and manufacturers during the design process. Antenna and RF solution providers need to know certain device requirements and will make sure the antenna it placed properly.

Government Support of Broadband for IoMT

Government agencies are recognizing the importance of broadband access to healthcare and are taking steps to improve access to broadband for medical purposes.

The FCC released a public notice seeking comments and data on actions to accelerate the adoption and accessibility of broadband-enabled healthcare solutions and advanced technologies. Enlarged wireless network technology will help improve patient care.

The document mentions that broadband networks are becoming more significant to the national wellbeing and that maximizing their availability will enable all Americans to take advantage of 21st-century healthcare.

The FCC is assisting in the adoption and accessibility of broadband enabled healthcare solutions, particularly in rural areas, by seeking information. The information will help the Commission identify specific areas where broadband connectivity is lacking.

Broadband continues to be a significant technology healthcare organizations need to embrace as they continue to deploy IoMT devices. Slower IT networks simply can't handle the strain of the increased traffic and are too restricting on movement. High-speed broadband allows devices to remain constantly and securely connected at all times so signals are transmitted correctly and effectively.

Healthcare organizations need to consider broadband connectivity as they design and deploy connected medical devices. As telemedicine programs grow, patients are dependent on device connectivity for their wellbeing.

Wi-Fi 6 Technology

Excerpts of an article from HIT Infrastructure:

Wi-Fi 6, 5G Could Be Turning Point for Health IT Infrastructure

Next-generation wireless networking technologies could be the solution to the proliferation of medical and mobile devices, which is threatening to overwhelm health IT infrastructure.

https://hitinfrastructure.com/features/wi-fi-6-5g-could-be-turning-point-for-health-it-infrastructure

Healthcare organizations are deploying more bandwidth-intensive connected medical devices and mobile devices, which are straining existing health IT infrastructure.

Next-generation wireless networking technologies, such as Wi-Fi 6 and 5G cellular, could be the solution to this growing problem.

To ease network congestion, the Wi-Fi 6 wireless networking standard is expected to provide higher data rates, increased capacity, strong performance with many connected devices, and improved power efficiency compared with present Wi-Fi versions.

Yet, the next generation of wireless technologies has certain issues that organizations need to consider. Upgrading to Wi-Fi 6 will involve significant investment in infrastructure and equipment.

What changes will Wi-Fi 6 bring?

The next-generation Wi-Fi 6 wireless networking standard could be a huge improvement for healthcare organizations operating many bandwidth-intensive connected devices.
In particular, Wi-Fi 6 offers:

- <u>Uplink and downlink orthogonal frequency division multiple access (OFDMA)</u>, which increases network efficiency and lowers latency for high-demand environments, such as hospitals
- <u>Multi-user multiple input multiple output (MU-MIMO)</u>, which allows more data to be transferred at the same time and enables an access point to transmit to a larger number of concurrent clients
- <u>Transmit beamforming</u>, which enables higher data rates at a given range resulting in greater network capacity
- <u>1024 quadrature amplitude modulation mode (1024-QAM)</u>, which increases throughput in Wi-Fi devices by encoding more data in the same amount of spectrum
- <u>Target wake time</u>, which improves battery life in Wi-Fi devices, such as Internet of Things devices

As part of the upgrade to Wi-Fi 6, the Wi-Fi Alliance adopted a new naming convention for Wi-Fi versions. Instead of having to remember 802.11ac, Wi-Fi users just need to remember Wi-Fi 5. For 802.11n, the designation is Wi-Fi 4.

And Wi-Fi 6 is based on the next-generation 802.11ax technology.

Wi-Fi 6 incorporates OFDMA, which increases network efficiency and lowers latency for high-demand networking environments.

With OFDMA, up to 30 devices can share a channel, rather than taking turns sending data. Wi-Fi 6-enabled wireless medical devices will work better, stay connected, and be more reliable, proponents say.

"From our perspective, Wi-Fi 6 is a fundamental change in the Wi-Fi ecosystem, because what we're doing is we're moving from OFDM to OFDMA, which means that there's some significant changes that are happening in this round," said Matt MacPherson, chief technology officer for Wireless at Cisco.

OFDMA is a multi-user version of OFDM, which is a method of encoding digital data on multiple carrier frequencies. In an OFDM system, the user or device is allocated on the time domain only, while in an OFDMA system the user or device is allocated on both time and frequency.

"With Wi-Fi, each device has a transmit opportunity, and it can send so much traffic in that transmit opportunity. Typically what it does is it sends a single stream of data," MacPherson told HITInfrastructure.com.

"In OFDMA, you can actually schedule in the frequency domain. This is new. What that means is that when you have a transmit opportunity, you can put multiple different streams of traffic into that transmit opportunity, so you're fully using it."

MacPherson described a scenario where doctors and nurses are using paging systems at the same time as Internet of Things devices, like heart monitors, are sending data. Wi-Fi 6 would give the organization the ability to prioritize that traffic so that the most important data is transmitted first.

"Wi-Fi 6 allows organizations to connect a lot more devices with much more consistent throughput. So not only is the individual throughput per device better, but also it's consistent across the network. Then as you add devices, that throughput will remain consistent, and it won't start to drop off," he explained.

Hospitals are an example of a congested, high-traffic environment that would benefit from other Wi-Fi 6 features, such as MU-MIMO, which enables an access point to transmit to a larger number of concurrent clients.

"The 8x8 MU-MIMO is going to be critical because that improves your overall spectral efficiency, being able to service eight clients at a time both on the uplink and downlink side," said Jay White, product manager of Wi-Fi products for Laird Connectivity.

Wi-Fi-enabled medical devices like infusion pumps can take advantage of scheduling-based resource allocation. Along with other devices and access points, the infusion pump can negotiate and define a specific time to send data.

"You also have things like target wake time. This will help with low-power medical devices that aren't in use 100 percent of the time. If they are running on a battery, they can stay asleep for longer durations of time and only wake up when it's critical for them to send data," White told HITInfrastructure.com.

"The real benefit to Wi-Fi 6 is improving the network efficiency as a whole, so the entire network gets lifted up by using Wi-Fi 6," White said.

Impediments to Upgrading to Wi-Fi 6

Wi-Fi 6 may offer strong technical advantages, but implementation might be delayed due to the cost of purchasing new hardware and the challenges of scheduling downtime in an organization that never takes a break.

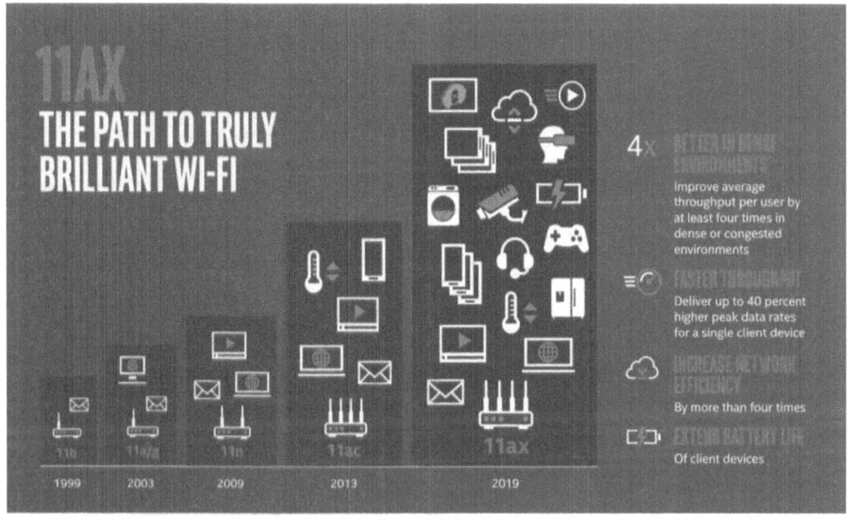

Overall, Wi-Fi 6 builds on 802.11ac with more than fifty updated features, though not all of them will necessarily be included in the finalized specification.

Here's some of what Wi-Fi 6 is expected to accomplish:

- More overall bandwidth per user for ultra-HD and virtual reality streaming
- Support for more simultaneous streams of data with increased throughput
- More total spectrum (2.4GHz and 5GHz, eventually bands in 1GHz and 6GHz)
- Said spectrum split into more channels to enable more routes for communication
- Packets contain more data and networks can handle different data streams at once
- Improved performance (as much as 4x) at the maximum range of an access point
- Better performance/robustness in outdoor and multi-path (cluttered) environments
- Ability to offload wireless traffic from cellular networks where reception is poor

Related Article:

Wi-Fi 6 Wireless Networking Standard Could Be Healthcare Game Changer

https://hitinfrastructure.com/news/wi-fi-6-wireless-networking-standard-could-be-healthcare-game-changer

WiFi 6 Vs 5G: What It Means for IoT

Excerpts of an article from IoT for All

New wireless standards are expected to revolutionize IoT, with blazing speeds, low power requirements and high bandwidth. As WiFi 6 and 5G hit the market in 2019, debates like "WiFi 6 vs 5G" for IoT will intensify.

https://www.iotforall.com/5g-vs-wifi6-iot-2019/

Written by Krystal Rogers-Nelson, Freelance Writer

Thanks to two new wireless standards rolling out this year—WiFi 6 and 5G—2019 is shaping up to be a watershed year for the Internet of Things (IoT). These new technologies are expected to revolutionize IoT, and mobile communications in general, with blazing speeds, low power requirements, and high bandwidth. Let's see what these emerging technologies are all about and why they're so exciting for the future of IoT

WiFi 6 Is More Than Just a Name

WiFi 6 is the name for the next generation of the wireless standard, following the current 802.11ac protocol. WiFi 6 is technically called 802.11ax, but in addition to new wireless technology, it's also bringing with it a new naming scheme: it'll be known simply as WiFi 6, while 802.11ac will be referred to as WiFi 5.

WiFi 6 will be up to four times faster in device-dense areas and offer much greater bandwidth than its predecessor. With internet service getting faster than ever, WiFi 6 will allow wireless devices to take full advantage of these new speeds.

These new technologies are expected to enable homes and businesses to have more devices active at once while using less energy. That's important, because experts predict nearly 31 billion installed IoT devices around the world by 2020.

5G Brings the Speed

5G is the name used for the next-gen cellular technology that will replace 4G LTE. Typically, cellular networks have covered larger areas, while WiFi handles things on a smaller scale. 5G may challenge this paradigm, though, with providers planning to offer personal 5G networks for in-home use.

5G cellular connections will be significantly faster than even the fastest LTE speeds currently available. Apart from faster speeds, 5G will bring much greater bandwidth and capacity to networks, just like WiFi 6. This will enable an explosion of devices as networks handle higher usage without a slowdown.

WiFi 6 and 5G Will Transform How We Use IoT Devices

Why all the fuss? Well, in addition to their faster speeds, both 5G and WiFi 6 will improve signal strength in congested areas, like downtown urban centers or crowded homes. These are places that previously had too much wireless traffic to make always-on devices practical, but with higher-capacity networks, this overcrowding problem will become a thing of the past.

On the business side, the new speed and bandwidth of WiFi 6 networks could be used to provide faster guest WiFi for customers and could also power connected devices like beacons to provide additional services to shoppers. The efficiency of the new technology could potentially lower costs on both networks and the devices themselves, enabling even small businesses to take advantage of these new technologies.

As another option, a 5G cellular connection could allow new business setups for connected devices. Retail store owners won't need to worry about connecting smart devices with multiple access points spread across different floors. Data-heavy devices like live security cameras won't eat up your bandwidth as they upload video.

On the consumer side, we may see not just a few specific devices but entire smart homes connected with 5G cellular rather than a home WiFi network. Many home security systems already use cellular networks for monitoring and reporting, but 5G can make it much simpler to install smart devices wherever you want. With future cellular devices, you could place your security cameras, smart locks, or digital assistants wherever there is 5G service instead of using Bluetooth, Z-Wave, or WiFi connections. 5G may also mean easier out-of-the-box setup because you won't need to configure devices to your WiFi.

How IoT Devices Will Change

As 5G and WiFi 6 come to the market in 2019, expect to see IoT devices designed to send more information and to use less power. These technologies could enable always-on, always-connected devices that use less energy and offer longer battery life.

Devices of all sorts are also likely to start shipping with SIM card trays or embedded SIM cards to enable the cellular functionality, which will be a change from the current trend of WiFi devices. WiFi won't go away entirely, but a long-range cellular connection offers a lot of advantages over a fixed WiFi network, especially when speeds are comparable. WiFi may become the fallback when 5G cellular isn't available, rather than the other way around as it currently is on many devices.

The rollout of WiFi 6 and especially 5G cellular networks will make 2019 a very exciting year for the IoT industry. While it's a little early to tell exactly how things will play out, one thing's for sure: there's a lot to look forward to.

5G Network Technology

The evolution of 5G wireless will enhance telemedicine and remote care by offering faster connections and higher bandwidths.

Healthcare organizations using advanced technology for telehealth and telemedicine care must consider the implications 5G technology will bring to the health infrastructure, especially as remote patient care and remote clinicians become more common.

The 5G wireless ecosystem is expected to expand in the near future due to the initiatives taken by national and regional governments with network providers and wireless carriers.

The evolution into 5G networking will allow users to get better connections on mobile devices, making Internet of Things (IoT) and remote devices more operational.

The 3rd Generation Partnership Project (3GPP) and other Standards Development Organizations (SDOs) are currently defining the first phase of 5G specifications before the first official 5G services are offered by vendors. The top wireless providers are rushing to be the first to offer standardized 5G services. Pre-Standard 5G networks are currently available in limited releases.

The 3GPP provides its organization partners with an environment to produce and test new telecommunication network standards that will form the basis of the global standard. The organization aims to help move the global mobile ecosystem from 4G LTE to a faster 5G deployment based on standards-compliant 5G NR infrastructure.

Many telemedicine programs currently rely on 4G technology to care for patients in remote areas, or patients who cannot leave their homes for treatment.

Some companies are offering reliable connectivity though 4G using a VPN to bring the information back to the data center in a way that is HIPAA compliant. They can perform many things they need to do over that medium-speed internet connection without relying on wires. Some early attempts tried to use patient in-home networks but it does not work reliably because there is a different environment in every home."

With the expected rollout of 5G technology, telemedicine programs will have faster, more reliable connections to the datacenter. The wider bandwidth will provide better video quality for conferencing and allow larger blocks of data to be transferred at a time.

Initial 5G services commenced in many countries in 2019 and widespread availability of 5G is expected by 2025.

Related Articles:
- 5G Explained http://www.emfexplained.info/?ID=25916

5G Wireless User Cases

Excerpts of an article from ZDNet:

What is 5G? The business guide to next-generation wireless technology

https://www.zdnet.com/article/what-is-5g-the-business-guide-to-next-generation-wireless-technology/

The most important promise made by the proprietors of 5G wireless technology -- the telecommunications service providers, the transmission equipment makers, the antenna manufacturers, and even the server manufacturers -- is this: Once all of 5G's components are fully deployed and operational, you will not need any kind of wire or cable to deliver communications or even entertainment service to your mobile device, to any of your fixed devices (HDTV, security system, smart appliances), or to your automobile. If everything works, 5G would be the optimum solution to the classic "last mile" problem: Delivering complete digital connectivity from the tip of the carrier network to the customer, without drilling another hole through the wall.

The "if" in that previous sentence remains colossal. The whole point of "Gs" in wireless standards, originally, was to emphasize the ease of transition between one wireless system of delivery and a newer one -- or at least make that transition seem reasonably pain-free.

User Cases

The revolution, like all others, will be subsidized. The initial costs of these 5G infrastructure improvements may be tremendous, and consumers have already demonstrated their intolerance for rate hikes. So to recover those costs, telcos will need to offer new classes of service to new customer segments, for which 5G has made provisions. Customers have to believe 5G wireless is capable of accomplishing feats that were impossible for 4G.

Driverless Automobiles. The autonomous vehicle (AV) use does expose one of the critical necessities of modern wireless infrastructure: It needs to connect people in motion with the computers they may be relying upon to save lives, with near-zero latency.

Explanation: The communications technology C-V2X, using the 5G networks, will allow vehicles to communicate wirelessly with each other, with traffic signals and with other roadside gear, improving both functionality and safety.

Virtual Reality (VR) and Augmented Reality (AR). For a cloud-based server to provide a believable, real-time sensory environment to a wireless user, as mobile processor maker Qualcomm asserted in a recent presentation, the connection between that server and its user may need to supply as much as 5 gigabits per second of bandwidth. In addition, the compute-intensive nature of an AR workload may actually mandate that such workloads be directed to servers stationed closer to their users, in systems that are relatively unencumbered by similar workloads being processed for other users. In other words, AR and VR may be better suited to small cell deployments anyway.

Cloud Computing. The internet is not just the conduit for content, but the facilitator of connectivity in wide-area networks (WAN). 5G wireless offers the potential for distributing cloud computing services much closer to users than most of Amazon's, Google's, or Microsoft's hyperscale data centers. In so doing, 5G could make telcos into competitors with these cloud providers, particularly for high-intensity, critical workloads. This is the edge computing scenario you may have heard about: Bringing processing power forward, closer to the customer, minimizing latencies caused by distance. If latencies can be eliminated just enough, applications that currently require PCs could be relocated to smaller devices -- perhaps even mobile devices that, unto themselves, have less processing power than the average smartphone.

Internet of Things. In a household with low-latency 5G connectivity, today's so-called "smart devices" that are essentially smartphone-class computers could be replaced with dumb terminals that get their instructions from nearby edge computing systems. Kitchen appliances, climate control systems, and more importantly, health monitors can all be made easier to produce and easier to control. The role played today by IoT hubs, which some manufacturers are producing today to cooperate alongside Wi-Fi routers, may in the future be played by 5G transmitters in the neighborhood, acting as service hubs for all the households in their coverage areas. In addition, machine-to-machine communications (M2M) enables scenarios where devices such as manufacturing robots can coordinate with one another for construction, assembly, and other tasks, under the collective guidance of an M2M hub at the 5G base station.

Healthcare. The availability of low-latency connectivity in rural areas would revolutionize critical care treatment for individuals nationwide. No longer would patients in small towns be forced to upend their lives and relocate to bigger cities, away from the livelihoods they know and love, just to receive the level of care to which they should be entitled. As recent trials in Mississippi are proving, connectivity at 5G levels enables caregivers in rural and remote areas to receive real-time instruction and support from the finest surgeons in the world, wherever they may be located.

To make the transition feasible in homes and businesses, telcos are looking to move customers into a 5G business track now, even before most true 5G services exist yet. More to the point, they're laying the "foundations" for technology tracks that can more easily be upgraded to 5G, once those 5G services do become available.

5G Explained – How 5G Works

Excerpts of the EMF Explained 2.0 website:

5G Explained   http://www.emfexplained.info/?ID=25916

WHAT IS 5G?

5G is the 5th generation of mobile networks, a significant evolution of todays 4G LTE networks. 5G has been designed to meet the very large growth in data and connectivity of today's modern society, the internet of things with billions of connected devices, and tomorrow's innovations. 5G will initially operate in conjunction with existing 4G networks before evolving to fully standalone networks in subsequent releases and coverage expansions.

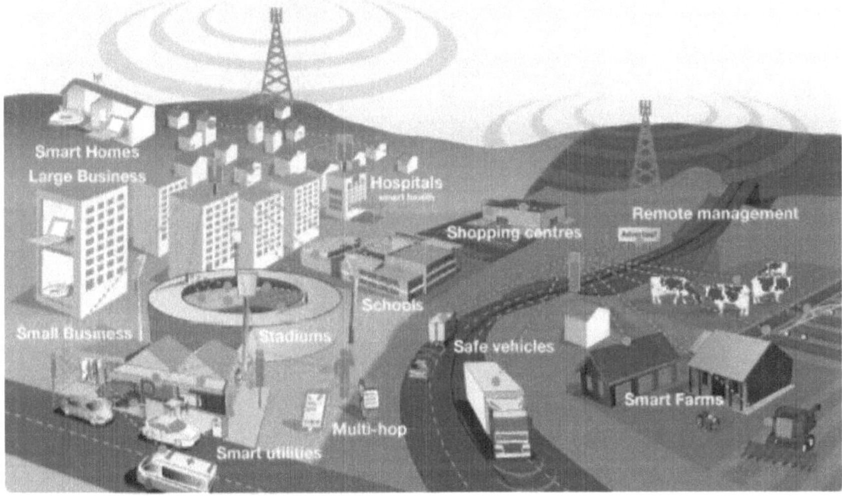

In addition to delivering faster connections and greater capacity, a very important advantage of 5G is the fast response time referred to as latency.

Latency is the time taken for devices to respond to each other over the wireless network. 3G networks had a typical response time of 100 milliseconds, 4G is around 30 milliseconds and 5G will be as low as 1 millisecond. This is virtually instantaneous opening up a new world of connected applications.

WHAT WILL 5G ENABLE?

5G will enable instantaneous connectivity to billions of devices, the Internet of Things (IoT) and a truly connected world.

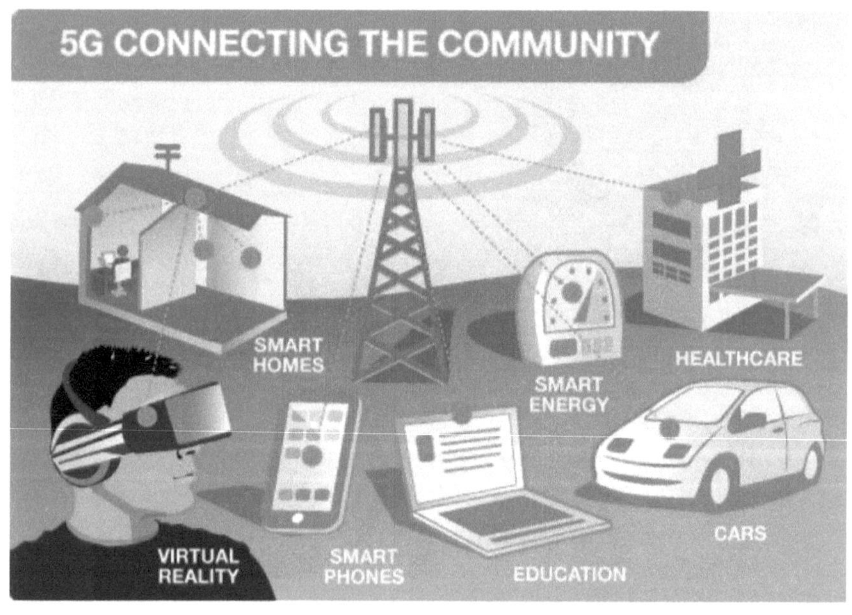

HOW DOES 5G WORK?

Most operators will initially integrate 5G networks with existing 4G networks to provide a continuous connection.

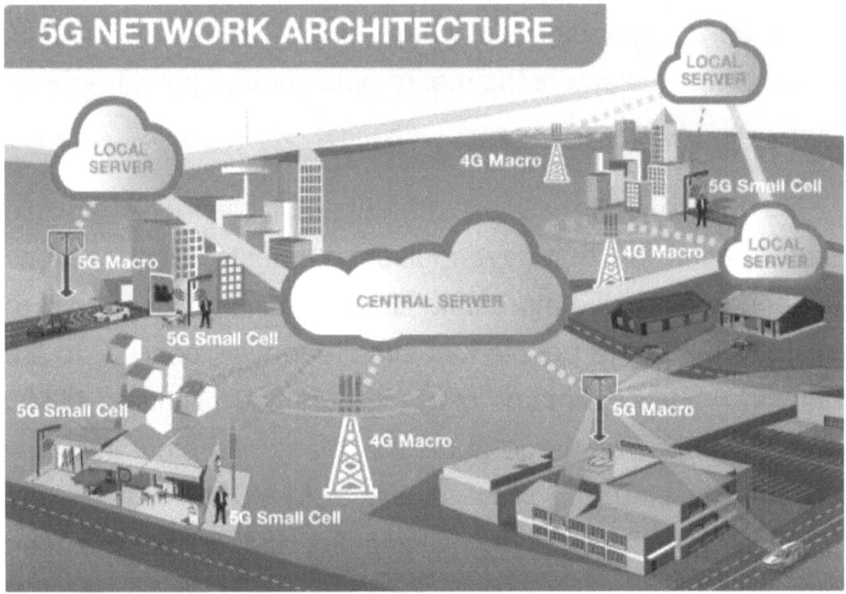

5G network architecture illustrating 5G and 4G working together, with central and local servers providing faster content to users and low latency applications.

A mobile network has two main components, the 'Radio Access Network' and the 'Core Network'.

The Radio Access Network - consists of various types of facilities including small cells, towers, masts and dedicated in-building and home systems that connect mobile users and wireless devices to the main core network.

Small cells will be a major feature of 5G networks particularly at the new millimeter wave (mmWave) frequencies where the connection range is very short. To provide a continuous connection, small cells will be distributed in clusters depending on where users require connection which will complement the macro network that provides wide-area coverage.

5G Macro Cells will use MIMO (multiple input, multiple output) antennas that have multiple elements or connections to send and receive more data simultaneously. The benefit to users is that more people can simultaneously connect to the network and maintain high throughput. Where MIMO antennas use very large numbers of antenna elements they are often referred to as 'massive MIMO', however, the physical size is similar to existing 3G and 4G base station antennas.

The Core Network - is the mobile exchange and data network that manages all of the mobile voice, data and internet connections. For 5G, the 'core network' is being redesigned to better integrate with the internet and cloud based services and also includes distributed servers across the network improving response times (reducing latency).

Many of the advanced features of 5G including network function virtualization and network slicing for different applications and services, will be managed in the core. The following illustration shows examples of local cloud servers providing faster content to users (movie streaming) and low latency applications for vehicle collision avoidance systems.

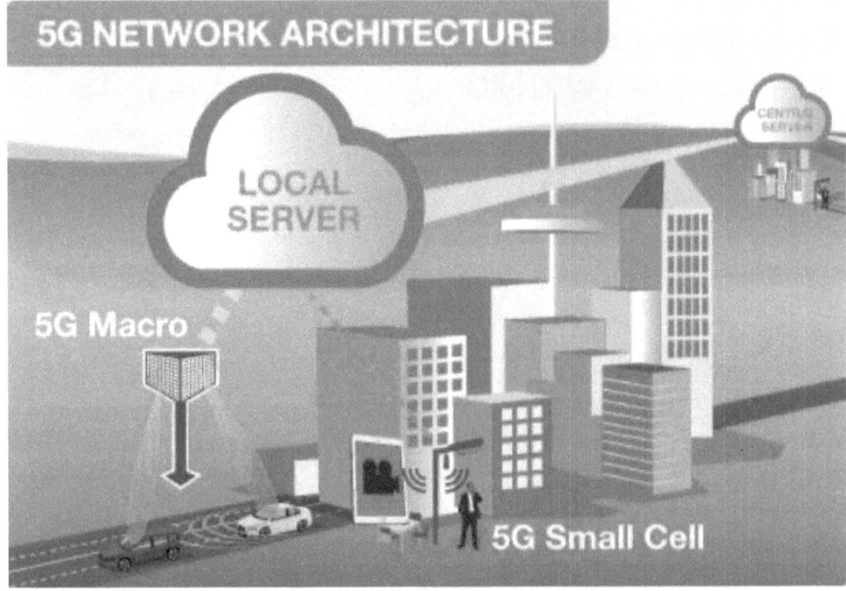

Example of a local server in a 5G network providing faster connection and lower response times.

Network Slicing – enables a smart way to segment the network for a particular industry, business or application. For example emergency services could operate on a network slice independently from other users.

Network Function Virtualization (NVF) - is the ability to instantiate network functions in real time at any desired location within the operator's cloud platform. Network functions that used to run on dedicated hardware for example a firewall and encryption at business premises can now operate on software on a virtual machine. NVF is crucial to enable the speed efficiency and agility to support new business applications and is an important technology for a 5G ready core.

5G WORKING WITH 4G

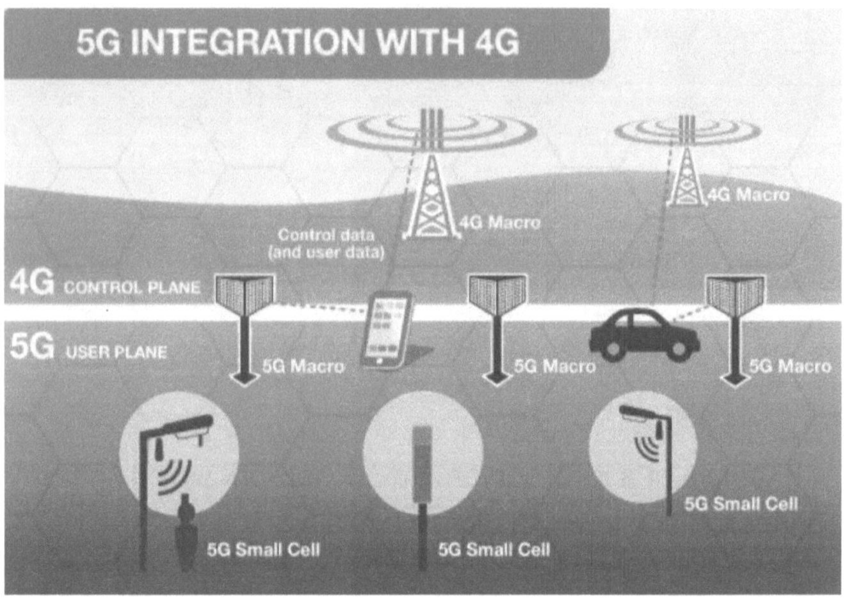

When a 5G connection is established, the User Equipment (or device) will connect to both the 4G network to provide the control signaling and to the 5G network to help provide the fast data connection by adding to the existing 4G capacity.

Where there is limited 5G coverage, the data is carried on the 4G network providing the continuous connection. Essentially with this design, the 5G network is complementing the existing 4G network

HOW DOES 5G DELIVER CONTINUOUS CONNECTION, GREATER CAPACITY, AND FASTER SPEED AND RESPONSE TIMES?

5G networks are designed to work in conjunction with 4G networks using a range of macro cells, small cells and dedicated in-building systems. Small cells are mini base stations designed for very localized coverage typically from 10 meters to a few hundred meters providing in-fill for a larger macro network. Small cells are essential for the 5G networks as the mmWave frequencies have a very short connection range.

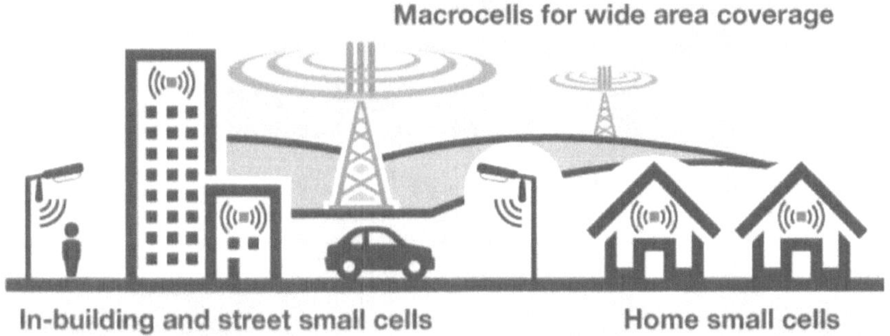

Increased Spectrum – Greater Capacity, More Users and Faster Speed

In many countries the initial frequency bands for 5G are below 6 GHz (in many cases in the 3.3-3.8 GHz bands) and similar frequencies to existing mobile and Wi-Fi networks. Additional mobile spectrum above 6 GHz, including the 26-28

GHz bands often referred to as millimeter (mm) Wave, will provide significantly more capacity compared to the current mobile technologies. The additional spectrum and greater capacity will enable more users, more data and faster connections. It is also expected that there will be future reuse of existing low band spectrum for 5G as legacy networks decline in usage and to support future use cases.

The increased spectrum in the mmWave band will provide localized coverage as they only operate over short distances. Future 5G deployments may use mmW frequencies in bands up to 86 GHz.

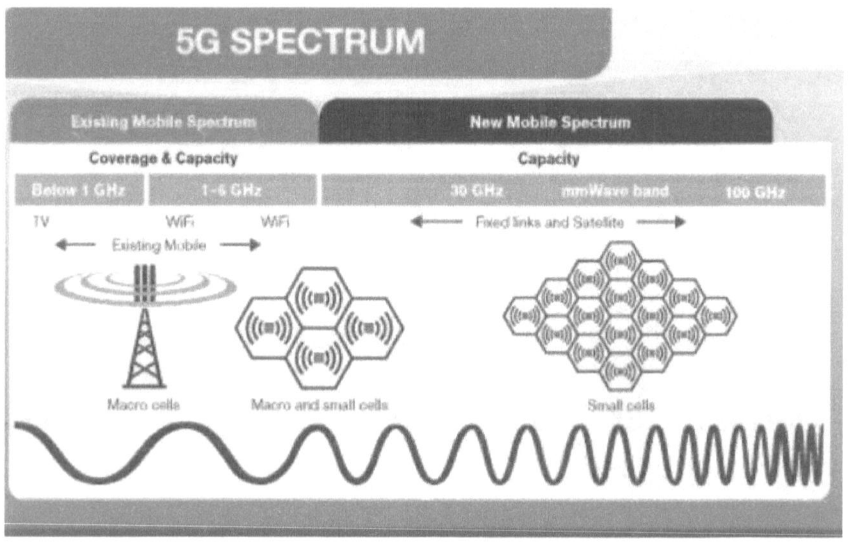

Mobile spectrum showing the radio frequency range from 3-100 GHz with new 5G spectrum above 6GHz.

Massive MIMO

Multiple element base station - greater capacity, multiple users, faster data

5G will use 'massive' MIMO (multiple input, multiple output) antennas that have very large numbers of antenna elements or connections to send and receive more data simultaneously. The benefit to users is that more people can simultaneously connect to the network and maintain high throughput.

The overall physical size of the 5G massive MIMO antennas will be similar to 4G, however with a higher frequency, the individual antenna element size is smaller allowing more elements (in excess of 100) in the same physical case.

5G User Equipment including mobile phones and devices will also have MIMO antenna technology built into the device for the mmWave frequencies.

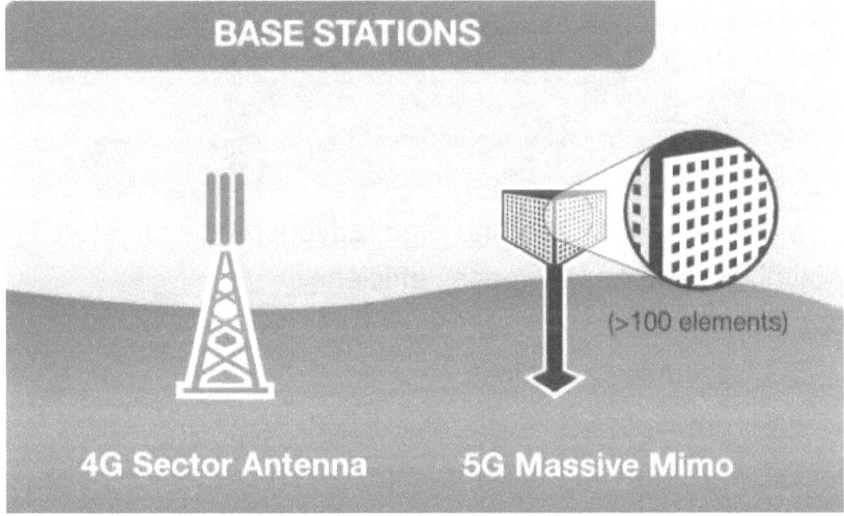

MIMO - Beam Steering

Beam steering is a technology that allows the massive MIMO base station antennas to direct the radio signal to the users and devices rather than in all directions. The beam steering technology uses advanced signal processing algorithms to determine the best path for the radio signal to reach the user. This increases efficiency as it reduces interference (unwanted radio signals).

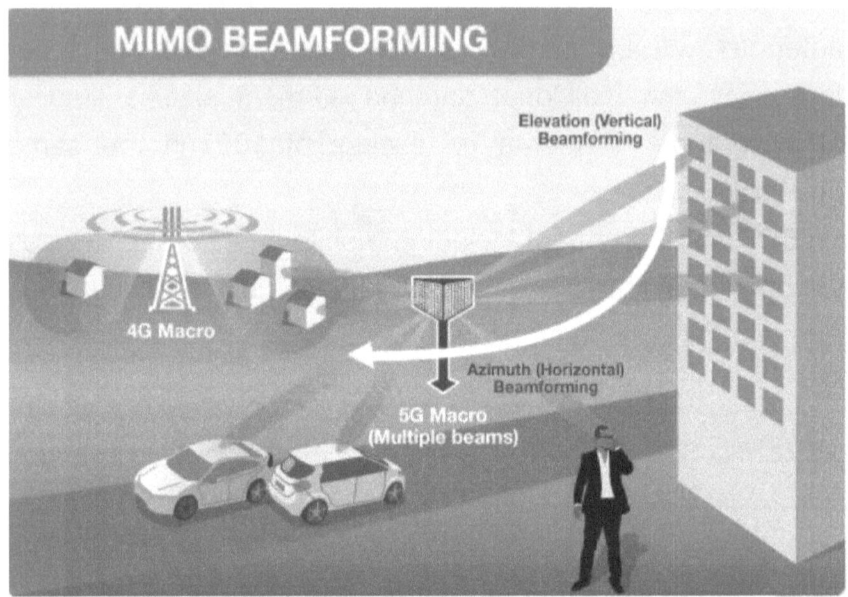

Massive MIMO antenna and advanced beam steering optimizes EMF and increases efficiency.

5G Resources and Links:

http://www.emfexplained.info/?ID=25915

http://www.emfexplained.info/?ID=24897

The Interoperability Challenge

Telemedicine's toughest problem, interoperability, is finally at an 'inflection point'.

The opportunities and challenges for healthcare stakeholders include standards, governance and workflows as telemedicine, which "has passed the tipping point of market momentum," gains traction nationwide, according to the ATA's report Telehealth Interoperability: Driving Choice, Continuity, and Scale.

The promise is immense, but big hurdles still remain before it reaches its full potential.

"In many cases, telemedicine clinical services and settings are fragmented and data is siloed, with low-volume telemedicine services such as those for specific locations or clinical specialties standing alone rather than being designed as part of a larger, integrated system," according to the ATA.

"As these fragmented systems proliferate, they result in costly, redundant software infrastructure and endpoints that limit the potential to improve overall quality and access to care," researchers wrote. "These fragmented systems also make it difficult for payers (government agencies, private insurers, and employers) to gain access to the comprehensive member data needed for claims and utilization management systems, and add to the challenges of performance tracking, reimbursement, and incentives."

Continuing to sort that out will require health systems to iron out some technical challenges related to telemedicine interoperability, which has some unique aspects related to patient ID, workflow, data capture, communication, regulatory issues and more.

And its specifications are also evolving as the technology and implementations mature. For example, when it comes to video conferencing, "robust standards including SIP/H323 exist but new options such as WEBRTC are making seamless connections possible in any browser without having to download additional apps. The industry can help evolve these standards and make medical devices work seamlessly as part of video conferences."

Interoperability is important for folks on both sides of the video screen, the ATA added.

"The patient experience will not be complete without integrated communication platforms to accompany the on-demand or scheduled telemedicine encounter," researchers write. "Interoperability must incorporate communication platforms across the gamut of secure paging, texting, IM, chats, video, phone/VOIP, faxing/e-faxing, and scanning. As standards, specifications, and interfaces become more robust and more broadly implemented, they will support an even richer telemedicine infrastructure and a seamless clinical experience."

The Larger Trend

Clearly, telemedicine's moment has arrived after 30 years of incremental progress, not just in the U.S., but worldwide. But for distance-based care to truly succeed, it needs to address many of the same interoperability questions that the rest of healthcare is grappling with in earnest.

And that's in addition to other sticking points, such as those outlined in a recent RAND report, which found that safety net providers – among those who most stand to benefit from telemedicine – are dealing with challenges related to infrastructure and broadband, cellular, technology costs, lack of buy-in among providers, complexities in adjusting clinic workflows and more.

On the Record

"Experienced health systems are defining near-term clinical requirements and connecting with like-minded technology vendors and payers," said ATA officials in the report. "Investments and aligned financial incentives are creating an environment to demonstrate the value of integrated clinical services that leverage interoperable platform technologies. And government and private payers, along with policy advocates, are working to increase incentives and favorable reimbursement models for broad-based telemedicine implementations to help drive continued improvements in cost, quality, and access."

"Interoperability of telemedicine will define its future," said Dr. Andrew Watson, president of the ATA and vice president of clinical information technology transformation at UPMC, in a statement. "In the era of value-based care, understanding data and how telemedicine relates to the frontline care systems of both payers and providers is critical. For telemedicine to be relevant – and even to be a frontline system itself – it must be interoperable for ease of use, cost of integration, security, and patient/member identification. This important interoperability initiative governs much of the promise for the future of telemedicine."

The ONC Awards Grants for Interoperability

The Office of the National Coordinator for Health Information Technology (ONC) has awarded grants to organizations in order to fund their work in improving healthcare interoperability.

The grants are being made under the Leading Edge Acceleration Projects in Health Information Technology (LEAP in Health IT) program, which is designed to advance the development and use of interoperable health IT.

https://hitinfrastructure.com/news/onc-ponies-up-close-to-2m-for-healthcare-interoperability-work

Big Data in Telemedicine

An inevitable piece of increased use of telemedicine is increased data collection. Frequency of visits, health outcomes, and population health statistics will all be better captured using telecommunications technology. So the natural next step in telemedicine is for telemedicine providers to begin analyzing and synthesizing the data they are collecting.

The data being collected has a lot of potential for enhancing care. Sophisticated analytics could be able to identify especially at-risk patients earlier on. The data could be used to develop more personalized treatment plans. It could predict acute medical events, such as heart failure. It could forecast disease outbreak. It could even do more mundane things, such as speed up insurance approvals and payment turnarounds. All of these could transform the medical industry, reducing costs and improving the quality of care.

While many consumers dislike the idea of their health data being collected, it is easy for companies to de-identify the data so that it can be analyzed without affecting patient privacy concerns. Big data has revolutionized many industries and allowed for better decision making. Health care could certainly be next. Big data allows for data-driven insights and trend analysis so that the medical community can be better informed and can deliver better care. If telemedicine technology providers can capitalize on the data they are collecting, they could evolve into true value drivers for the entire health care system.

The question is how this piece of the industry will develop. Will telemedicine companies partner with big data companies to analyze their data? Or will telemedicine companies develop their own sophisticated data and analytics teams within? Either way, big data collected by telemedicine could lead to new insights and advances in health care.

Conclusion

There are many roads telemedicine could take in the future. As more and more people become familiar with technology and comfortable using it in their everyday lives, use of telemedicine will advance. Different experts and different companies have differing and sometimes competing visions for the future of telemedicine. While they may not all develop as they think, it is exciting to see and hear the potential of telemedicine technologies for the future of healthcare. It does seem that health care is often the last industry to embrace innovations, but that is only natural given that health is so important and personal. More companies are starting to push the envelope on how technology can improve access and communication in health care. And as a new generation of physicians develops that grew up with technology and a connected world, more and more medical facilities will embrace the innovations.

Artificial Intelligence in Healthcare

Healthcare's big data concentrated nature makes artificial intelligence an ideal candidate for the application across multiple disciplines, from diagnosis and pathology to drug discovery and epidemiology.

Article in HEALTH IT ANALYTICS:

Top 12 Ways Artificial Intelligence Will Impact Healthcare

https://healthitanalytics.com/news/top-12-ways-artificial-intelligence-will-impact-healthcare

The healthcare industry is ripe for some major changes. From chronic diseases and cancer to radiology and risk assessment, there are nearly endless opportunities to leverage technology to deploy more precise, efficient, and impactful interventions at exactly the right moment in a patient's care.

As payment structures evolve, patients demand more from their providers, and the volume of available data continues to increase at a staggering rate, artificial intelligence is poised to be the engine that drives improvements across the care continuum.

AI offers a number of advantages over traditional analytics and clinical decision-making techniques. Learning algorithms can become more precise and accurate as they interact with training data, allowing humans to gain unprecedented insights into diagnostics, care processes, treatment variability, and patient outcomes.

At the 2018 World Medical Innovation Forum (WMIF) on artificial intelligence presented by Partners Healthcare, a leading researchers and clinical faculty members showcased the twelve technologies and areas of the healthcare industry that are most likely to see a major impact from artificial intelligence within the next decade.

Every member of this "Disruptive Dozen" has the potential to produce a significant benefit to patients while possessing the potential for broad commercial success, said WMIF co-chairs Anne Kiblanksi, MD, Chief Academic Officer at Partners Healthcare and Gregg Meyer, MD, Chief Clinical Officer.

With the help of experts from across the Partners Healthcare system, including faculty from Harvard Medical School (HMS), moderators Keith Dreyer, DO, PhD, Chief Data Science Officer at Partners and Katherine Andriole, PhD, Director of Research Strategy and Operations at Massachusetts General Hospital (MGH), counted down the top 12 ways artificial intelligence will revolutionize the delivery and science of healthcare.

UNIFYING MIND AND MACHINE THROUGH BRAIN-COMPUTER INTERFACES

Using computers to communicate is not a new idea by any means, but creating direct interfaces between technology and the human mind without the need for keyboards, mice, and monitors is a cutting-edge area of research that has significant applications for some patients.

Neurological diseases and trauma to the nervous system can take away some patients' abilities to speak, move, and interact meaningfully with people and their environments. Brain-computer interfaces (BCIs) backed by artificial intelligence could restore those fundamental experiences to those who feared them lost forever.

"If I'm in the neurology ICU on a Monday, and I see someone who has suddenly lost the ability to move or to speak, we want to restore that ability to communicate by Tuesday," said Leigh Hochberg, MD, PhD, Director of the Center for Neurotechnology and Neurorecovery at MGH.

"By using a BCI and artificial intelligence, we can decode the neural activates associated with the intended movement of one's hand, and we should be able to allow that person to communicate the same way as many people in this room have communicated at least five times over the course of the morning using a ubiquitous communication technology like a tablet computer or phone."

Brain-computer interfaces could drastically improve quality of life for patients with ALS, strokes, or locked-in syndrome, as well as the 500,000 people worldwide who experience spinal cord injuries every year.

DEVELOPING THE NEXT GENERATION OF RADIOLOGY TOOLS

Radiological images obtained by MRI machines, CT scanners, and x-rays offer non-invasive visibility into the inner workings of the human body. But many diagnostic processes still rely on physical tissue samples obtained through biopsies, which carry risks including the potential for infection.

Artificial intelligence will enable the next generation of radiology tools that are accurate and detailed enough to replace the need for tissue samples in some cases, experts predict.

"We want to bring together the diagnostic imaging team with the surgeon or interventional radiologist and the pathologist," said Alexandra Golby, MD, Director of Image-Guided Neurosurgery at Brigham & Women's Hospital (BWH). "That coming together of different teams and aligning goals is a big challenge."

"If we want the imaging to give us information that we presently get from tissue samples, then we're going to have to be able to achieve very close registration so that the ground truth for any given pixel is known."

Succeeding in this quest may allow clinicians to develop a more accurate understanding of how tumors behave as a whole instead of basing treatment decisions on the properties of a small segment of the malignancy.

Providers may also be able to better define the aggressiveness of cancers and target treatments more appropriately.

Artificial intelligence is helping to enable "virtual biopsies" and advance the innovative field of radiomics, which focuses on harnessing image-based algorithms to characterize the phenotypes and genetic properties of tumors.

EXPANDING ACCESS TO CARE IN UNDERSERVED OR DEVELOPING REGIONS

Shortages of trained healthcare providers, including ultrasound technicians and radiologists can significantly limit access to life-saving care in developing nations around the world.

More radiologists work in the half-dozen hospitals lining the renowned Longwood Avenue in Boston than in all of West Africa, the session pointed out.

Artificial intelligence could help mitigate the impacts of this severe deficit of qualified clinical staff by taking over some of the diagnostic duties typically allocated to humans.

For example, AI imaging tools can screen chest x-rays for signs of tuberculosis, often achieving a level of accuracy comparable to humans. This capability could be deployed through an app available to providers in low-resource areas, reducing the need for a trained diagnostic radiologist on site.

"The potential for this tech to increase access to healthcare is tremendous," said Jayashree Kalpathy-Cramer, PhD, Assistant in Neuroscience at MGH and Associate Professor of Radiology at HMS.

However, algorithm developers must be careful to account for the fact that disparate ethnic groups or residents of different regions may have unique physiologies and environmental factors that will influence the presentation of disease.

"The course of a disease and population affected by the disease may look very different in India than in the US, for example," she said.

"As we're developing these algorithms, it's very important to make sure that the data represents a diversity of disease presentations and populations – we can't just develop an algorithm based on a single population and expect it to work as well on others."

REDUCING THE BURDENS OF ELECTRONIC HEALTH RECORD USE

EHRs have played an instrumental role in the healthcare industry's journey towards digitalization, but the switch has brought myriad problems associated with cognitive overload, endless documentation, and user burnout.

EHR developers are now using artificial intelligence to create more intuitive interfaces and automate some of the routine processes that consume so much of a user's time.

"Users spend the majority of their time on three tasks: clinical documentation, order entry, and sorting through the in-basket", said Adam Landman, MD, Vice President and CIO at Brigham Health.

Voice recognition and dictation are helping to improve the clinical documentation process, but natural language processing (NLP) tools might not be going far enough.

"I think we may need to be even bolder and consider changes like video recording a clinical encounter, almost like police wear body cams," said Landman. "And then you can use AI and machine learning to index those videos for future information retrieval."

"And just like in the home, where we're using Siri and Alexa, the future will bring virtual assistants to the bedside for clinicians to use with embedded intelligence for order entry."

Artificial intelligence may also help to process routine requests from the inbox, like medication refills and result notifications. It may also help to prioritize tasks that truly require the clinician's attention, Landman added, making it easier for users to work through their to-do lists.

CONTAINING THE RISKS OF ANTIBIOTIC RESISTANCE

Antibiotic resistance is a growing threat to populations around the world as overuse of these critical drugs fosters the evolution of superbugs that no longer respond to treatments. Multi-drug resistant organisms can wreak havoc in the hospital setting, and claim thousands of lives every year.

C.-difficile alone accounts for approximately $5 billion in annual costs for the US healthcare system and claims more than 30,000 lives.

Electronic health record data can help to identify infection patterns and highlight patients at risk before they begin to show symptoms. Leveraging machine learning and AI tools to drive these analytics can enhance their accuracy and create faster, more accurate alerts for healthcare providers.

"AI tools can live up to the expectation for infection control and antibiotic resistance," Erica Shenoy, MD, PhD, Associate Chief of the Infection Control Unit at MGH.

"If they don't, then that's really a failure on all of our parts. For the hospitals sitting on mountains of EHR data and not using them to the fullest potential, to industry that's not creating smarter, faster clinical trial design, and for EHRs that are creating these data not to use them…that would be a failure."

CREATING MORE PRECISE ANALYTICS FOR PATHOLOGY IMAGES

"Pathologists provide one of the most significant sources of diagnostic data for providers across the spectrum of care delivery", says Jeffrey Golden, MD, Chair of the Department of Pathology at BWH and a professor of pathology at HMS.

"Seventy percent of all decisions in healthcare are based on a pathology result," he said. "Somewhere between 70 and 75 percent of all the data in an EHR are from a pathology result. So the more accurate we get, and the sooner we get to the right diagnosis, the better we're going to be. That's what digital pathology and AI has the opportunity to deliver."

Analytics that can drill down to the pixel level on extremely large digital images can allow providers to identify nuances that may escape the human eye.

"We're now getting to the point where we can do a better job of assessing whether a cancer is going to progress rapidly or slowly and how that might change how patients will be treated based on an algorithm rather than clinical staging or the histopathologic grade," said Golden. "That's going to be a huge advance."

Artificial intelligence can also improve productivity by identifying features of interest in slides before a human clinician reviews the data, he added.

"AI can screen through slides and direct us to the right thing to look at so we can assess what's important and what's not. That increases the efficiency of the use of the pathologist and increases the value of the time they spend for each case."

BRINGING INTELLIGENCE TO MEDICAL DEVICES AND MACHINES

Smart devices are taking over the consumer environment, offering everything from real-time video from the inside of a refrigerator to cars that can detect when the driver is distracted.

In the medical environment, smart devices are critical for monitoring patients in the ICU and elsewhere. Using artificial intelligence to enhance the ability to identify deterioration, suggest that sepsis is taking hold, or sense the development of complications can significantly improve outcomes and may reduce costs related to hospital-acquired condition penalties.

"When we're talking about integrating disparate data from across the healthcare system, integrating it, and generating an alert that would alert an ICU doctor to intervene early on – the aggregation of that data is not something that a human can do very well," said Mark Michalski, MD, Executive Director of the MGH & BWH Center for Clinical Data Science.

Inserting intelligent algorithms into these devices can reduce cognitive burdens for physicians while ensuring that patients receive care in as timely a manner as possible.

ADVANCING THE USE OF IMMUNOTHERAPY FOR CANCER TREATMENT

Immunotherapy is one of the most promising avenues for treating cancer. By using the body's own immune system to attack malignancies, patients may be able to beat stubborn tumors. However, only a small number of patients respond to current immunotherapy options, and oncologists still do not have a precise and reliable method for identifying which patients will benefit from this option.

Machine learning algorithms and their ability to synthesize highly complex datasets may be able to illuminate new options for targeting therapies to an individual's unique genetic makeup.

"Recently, the most exciting development has been checkpoint inhibitors, which block some of the proteins made by some types of immune cells," explained Long Le, MD, PhD, Director of Computational Pathology and Technology Development at the MGH Center for Integrated Diagnostics. "But we still don't understand all of the disease biology. This is a very complex problem."

"We definitely need more patient data. The therapies are relatively new, so not a lot of patients have actually been put on these drugs. So whether we need to integrate data within one institution or across multiple institutions is going to be a key factor in terms of augmenting the patient population to drive the modeling process."

TURNING THE ELECTRONIC HEALTH RECORD INTO A RELIABLE RISK PREDICTOR

EHRs are a goldmine of patient data, but extracting and analyzing that wealth of information in an accurate, timely, and reliable manner has been a continual challenge for providers and developers.

Data quality and integrity issues, plus a mishmash of data formats, structured and unstructured inputs, and incomplete records have made it very difficult to understand exactly how to engage in meaningful risk stratification, predictive analytics, and clinical decision support.

"Part of the hard work is integrating the data into one place," observed Ziad Obermeyer, MD, Assistant Professor of Emergency Medicine at BWH and Assistant Professor at HMS. "But another problem is understanding what it is you're getting when you're predicting a disease in an EHR."

"You might hear that an algorithm can predict depression or stroke, but when you scratch the surface, you find what they're actually predicting is a billing code for stroke. That's very different from stroke itself."

"Relying on MRI results might appear to offer a more concrete dataset", he continued.

"But now you have to think about who can afford the MRI, and who can't? So what you end up predicting isn't what you thought you were predicting. You might be predicting billing for a stroke in people who can pay for a diagnostic rather than some sort of cerebral ischemia."

EHR analytics have produced many successful risk scoring and stratification tools, especially when researchers employ deep learning techniques to identify novel connections between seemingly unrelated datasets.

But ensuring that those algorithms do not confirm hidden biases in the data is crucial for deploying tools that will truly improve clinical care, Obermeyer maintained.

"The biggest challenge will be making sure exactly what we're predicting even before we start opening up the black box and looking at how we're predicting it," he said.

MONITORING HEALTH THROUGH WEARABLES AND PERSONAL DEVICES

Almost all consumers now have access to devices with sensors that can collect valuable data about their health. From smartphones with step trackers to wearables that can track a heartbeat around the clock, a growing proportion of health-related data is generated on the go.

Collecting and analyzing this data – and supplementing it with patient-provided information through apps and other home monitoring devices – can offer a unique perspective into individual and population health.

Artificial intelligence will play a significant role in extracting actionable insights from this large and varied treasure trove of data.

"But helping patients get comfortable with sharing data from this intimate, continual monitoring may require a little extra work", says Omar Arnaout, MD, Co-director of the Computation Neuroscience Outcomes Center and an attending neurosurgeon at BWH.

"As a society, we've been pretty liberal with our digital data," he said. But as things come into our collective consciousness like Cambridge Analytica and Facebook, people will become more and more prudent about who they share what kinds of data with."

However, patients tend to trust their physicians more than they might trust a big company like Facebook, he added, which may help to ease any discomfort with contributing data to large-scale research initiatives.

"There's a very good chance [wearable data will have a major impact] because our care is very episodic and the data we collect is very coarse," said Arnaout. "By collecting granular data in a continuous fashion, there's a greater likelihood that the data will help us take better care of patients."

MAKING SMARTPHONE SELFIES INTO POWERFUL DIAGNOSTIC TOOLS

Continuing the theme of harnessing the power of portable devices, experts believe that images taken from smartphones and other consumer-grade sources will be an important supplement to clinical quality imaging – especially in underserved populations or developing nations.

The quality of cell phone cameras is increasing every year, and can produce images that are viable for analysis by artificial intelligence algorithms. Dermatology and ophthalmology are early beneficiaries of this trend.

Researchers in the United Kingdom have even developed a tool that identifies developmental diseases by analyzing images of a child's face. The algorithm can detect discrete features, such as a child's jaw line, eye and nose placement, and other attributes that might indicate a craniofacial abnormality. Currently, the tool can match the ordinary images to more than 90 disorders to provide clinical decision support.

"The majority of the population is equipped with pocket-sized, powerful devices that have a lot of different sensors built in," said Hadi Shafiee, PhD, Director of the Laboratory of Micro/Nanomedicine and Digital Health at BWH.

"This is a great opportunity for us. Almost every major player in the industry has started to build AI software and hardware into their devices. That's not a coincidence. Every day in our digital world, we generate more than 2.5 million terabytes of data. In cell phones, the manufacturers believe they can use that data with AI to provide much more personalized and faster and smarter services."

Using smartphones to collect images of eyes, skin lesions, wounds, infections, medications, or other subjects may be able to help underserved areas cope with a shortage of specialists while reducing the time-to-diagnosis for certain complaints.

"There is something big happening," said Shafiee. "We can leverage that opportunity to address some of the important problems with have in disease management at the point of care."

REVOLUTIONIZING CLINICAL DECISION MAKING WITH ARTIFICIAL INTELLIGENCE AT THE BEDSIDE

As the healthcare industry shifts away from fee-for-service, so too is it moving further and further from reactive care. Getting ahead of chronic diseases, costly acute events, and sudden deterioration is the goal of every provider – and reimbursement structures are finally allowing them to develop the processes that will enable proactive, predictive interventions.

Artificial intelligence will provide much of the bedrock for that evolution by powering predictive analytics and clinical decision support tools that clue providers in to problems long before they might otherwise recognize the need to act.

AI can provide earlier warnings for conditions like seizures or sepsis, which often require intensive analysis of highly complex datasets.

"Machine learning can also help support decisions around whether or not to continue care for critically ill patients, such as those who have entered a coma after cardiac arrest", says

Brandon Westover, MD, PhD, Director of the MGH Clinical Data Animation Center.

"Typically, providers must visually inspect EEG data from these patients", he explained. The process is time-consuming and subjective, and the results may vary with the skill and experience of the individual clinician.

"In these patients, trends might be slowly evolving," he said. "Sometimes when we're looking to see if someone is recovering, we take the data from ten seconds of monitoring at a time. But trying to see if it changed from ten seconds of data taken 24 hours ago is like trying to look if your hair is growing longer."

"But if you have an AI algorithm and lots and lots of data from many patients, it's easier to match up what you're seeing to long term patterns and maybe detect subtle improvements that would impact your decisions around care."

Leveraging AI for clinical decision support, risk scoring, and early alerting is one of the most promising areas of development for this revolutionary approach to data analysis.

By powering a new generation of tools and systems that make clinicians more aware of nuances, more efficient when delivering care, and more likely to get ahead of developing problems, AI will usher in a new era of clinical quality and exciting breakthroughs in patient care.

AI-assisted Diagnosis

Artificial Intelligence (AI) is revolutionizing medical diagnostics with its learning skills. The result is that some AI programs can detect patterns better than human eyes.

It paves the way for the emergence of a new generation of medical diagnostic devices that can surpass the detection capabilities of the best physicians.

Since AI can be replicated, the expertise of these systems can be made available to a large number of patients.

Moreover, AI has many and diverse applications in medical diagnostics, such as image analysis for tumor detection, video detection for gait disorders and fall prediction, biochemical tests such as for diabetes or speech analysis of emotional state and psychiatric disorders. Therefore, the AI will significantly disrupt the traditional model of medical diagnosis.

AI Can also Assist Primary Care Physicians

For artificial intelligence, health care is the new frontier of research and development. Surgeons routinely use robot assistants to work less invasively and more accurately. Also, gene sequencing and gene editing aided by AI is changing the way scientists obtain cures for diseases.

In particular, however, research is being conducted so that AI can change the way physicians diagnose patients.

Envision the following Online Diagnosis Procedure:

Picture this situation for **a person fitted with a Health Armband** that continuously monitors vital signs such as respiratory rate, oxygen levels, pulse, blood pressure, and body temperature, **and is also equipped with a Home Medical Exam Kit** that includes an exam camera, a basal thermometer, an otoscope, a stethoscope and tongue depressor adapters. These HIPAA-secure digital devices transmit results to an electronic health record.

- You have symptoms of a cold. But, your fever hasn't subsided in days. You also experience occasionally a shortness of breath. You access the telemedicine app on your smart phone and make a video call.
- The doctor in his practice or clinic / hospital will ask you for your symptoms and records them on his Tablet **while watching you (via your exam camera) and your online Health Armband and Exam Kit data in real time**.
- Within seconds, an AI diagnosis system pulls up all your medical history and your on-line real-time data, puts your symptoms (entered by the doctor) into the context of your medical info, then gives the doctor a recommendation of the diagnosis.
- The doctor looks over the diagnosis and compares it with his/her personal evaluation.
- Then, the doctor discusses this diagnosis with you and the prescription is forwarded to your pharmacy.

AI facial recognition safeguards the conversation. You do not need to travel and you avoid waiting in the doctor's office or clinic. This is the future of medical diagnosis - an AI diagnostic system that helps doctors diagnose all kinds of diseases.

The AI vital signs processing could also have been configured to **automatically** alert the doctor of the condition and have him call the patient – a predictive health deterioration analysis.

Medical History:

Telemedicine programs often entail a comprehensive physical examination first and then follow-up routine physicals to update the patient's Medical History.

Comprehensive Physical (from Wikipedia)

Comprehensive physical exams, also known as executive physicals, typically include laboratory tests, chest x-rays, pulmonary function testing, audiograms, full body CAT scanning, EKGs, heart stress tests, vascular age tests, urinalysis, and mammograms or prostate exams depending on gender.

Routine Physicals (from Wikipedia)

The routine physical, also known as general medical examination is a physical examination performed on an asymptomatic patient for medical screening purposes. These are normally performed by a pediatrician, family practice physician, physician assistant, a certified nurse practitioner or other primary care provider. This routine physical exam usually includes the HEENT evaluation. Nursing professionals such as Registered Nurse, Licensed Practical Nurses can develop a baseline assessment to identify normal versus abnormal findings. These are reported to the primary care provider. If necessary, the patient may be sent to a medical specialist for further, more detailed examinations.

The general medical examination typically involves a medical history, a (brief or complete) physical examination and sometimes laboratory tests. Some more advanced tests include ultrasound and mammography.

Note: The above does **not** signify an exam recommendation.

The Technology Behind AI for Diagnosis

The artificial intelligence (AI) systems for diagnosis use deep learning techniques to arrive at a diagnosis. The systems source image data and symptoms data from healthcare facilities to train on, then, the systems use the techniques to arrive at the diagnosis.

The problem with deep learning techniques is transparency. Although the inputs and the outputs to the artificial intelligence systems are transparent, the way in which the simulated intelligence systems arrive at the diagnosis decision is often unclear

In addition, the AI system relies on the quality of the data to ensure accuracy.

Challenges in Data Collection

In the U.S., healthcare data is located in various healthcare facilities, at insurance companies, and inside government agencies. Obtaining all of the data into a data cloud for artificial intelligence systems to use is a daunting task. Businesses are currently embarked on building the exact infrastructure for medical technology and healthcare facilities to use to train their artificial intelligence systems. It is a significant investment for companies to go through all the regulations and privacy policies to provide this infrastructure.

Apart from these challenges, the future of artificial intelligence in medical diagnosis looks promising.

Medical Imaging

One of the areas in which artificial intelligence systems can be used both to automate the workflow and to aid diagnosis is Medical Imaging.

Medical images such as x-rays, ultrasound, CT or MRI images can be used to diagnose a variety of diseases. Radiologists are currently reviewing such scans for diagnosis. Depending on image quality, radiologists may often make mistakes due to limitations of the human eye or lack of experience in a particular disease area. Reviewing the images often takes time.

In the emergency department, a time-critical review of the images can lead to life-saving results.

An AI system can use its "extended view" to scan medical images for anomalies. Based on the training data, the AI system can detect these abnormalities and submit them to the radiologist for review. In addition, autonomous AI systems can efficiently diagnose diseases that clearly identify their unique causes for the AI system.

The repetitive work of reviewing the scans to look for abnormalities is automated. Once the abnormalities are identified, radiologists can use their experience to make the diagnosis.

The improved efficiency in the radiology workflow leads to a more accurate and a faster diagnosis.

Conclusion

As artificial intelligence innovations progress in healthcare, it is critical for medical device companies, data providers, hospitals, governments and insurance companies to work together to foster an atmosphere of innovation. In this innovation atmosphere better possibilities for the automation can be determined and appropriate data can be sourced, thus leading to better accuracy in both medical diagnosis and better efficiency in the healthcare workflow.

However, artificial intelligence will only be assistive and will not replace healthcare professionals in the near future. Today's potential is to have a computer algorithm that helps doctors with difficult diagnoses.

The Future: AI-assisted Diagnosis with Cause and Action Display

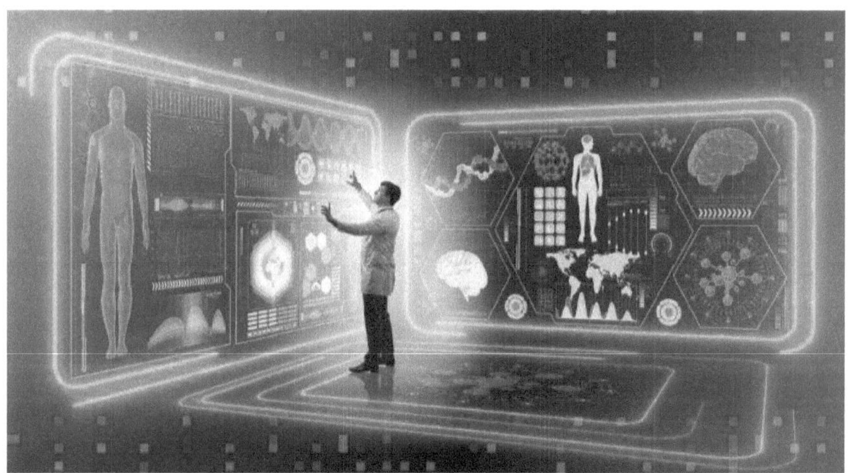

Genetic Testing (DNA Examination)

For scientists, the future is medical data - vast amounts of data. They examine your genome for risk factors and track tens of thousands of molecules that are active in your body.

In this way, the doctors of the future can identify and treat diseases long before symptoms appear.

However, the approach has a number of critics, who say it will instead lead to overtreatment of anxious patients.

The following is an article from the MAYO CLINIC:

Overview

Genetic testing involves examining your DNA, the chemical database that carries instructions for your body's functions. Genetic testing can reveal changes (mutations) in your genes that may cause illness or disease.

Although genetic testing can provide important information for diagnosing, treating and preventing illness, there are limitations. For example, if you're a healthy person, a positive result from genetic testing doesn't always mean you will develop a disease. On the other hand, in some situations, a negative result doesn't guarantee that you won't have a certain disorder.

Talking to your doctor, a medical geneticist or a genetic counselor about what you will do with the results is an important step in the process of genetic testing.

Genome Sequencing

When genetic testing doesn't lead to a diagnosis but a genetic cause is still suspected, some facilities offer genome sequencing — a process for analyzing a sample of DNA taken from your blood.

Everyone has a unique genome, made up of the DNA in all of a person's genes. This complex testing can help identify genetic variants that may relate to your health. This testing is usually limited to just looking at the protein-encoding parts of DNA called the exome.

Why It's Done

Genetic testing plays a vital role in determining the risk of developing certain diseases as well as screening and sometimes medical treatment. Different types of genetic testing are done for different reasons:

- **Diagnostic testing**. If you have symptoms of a disease that may be caused by genetic changes, sometimes called mutated genes, genetic testing can reveal if you have the suspected disorder. For example, genetic testing may be used to confirm a diagnosis of cystic fibrosis or Huntington's disease.

- **Presymptomatic and predictive testing**. If you have a family history of a genetic condition, getting genetic testing before you have symptoms may show if you're at risk of developing that condition. For example, this type of test may be useful for identifying your risk of certain types of colorectal cancer.

- **Carrier testing**. If you have a family history of a genetic disorder — such as sickle cell anemia or cystic fibrosis — or you're in an ethnic group that has a high risk of a specific genetic disorder, you may choose to have genetic testing before having children. An expanded carrier screening test can detect genes associated with a wide variety of genetic diseases and mutations and can identify if you and your partner are carriers for the same conditions.

- **Pharmacogenetics**. If you have a particular health condition or disease, this type of genetic testing may help determine what medication and dosage will be most effective and beneficial for you.

- **Prenatal testing**. If you're pregnant, tests can detect some types of abnormalities in your baby's genes. Down syndrome and trisomy 18 syndrome are two genetic disorders that are often screened for as part of prenatal genetic testing. Traditionally this is done looking at markers in blood or by invasive testing such as amniocentesis. Newer testing called cell-free DNA testing looks at a baby's DNA via a blood test done on the mother.

- **Newborn screening**. This is the most common type of genetic testing. In the United States, all states require that newborns be tested for certain genetic and metabolic abnormalities that cause specific conditions. This type of genetic testing is important because if results show there's a disorder such as congenital hypothyroidism, sickle cell disease or phenylketonuria (PKU), care and treatment can begin right away.

- **Preimplantation testing**. Also called preimplantation genetic diagnosis, this test may be used when you attempt to conceive a child through in vitro fertilization. The embryos are screened for genetic abnormalities. Embryos without abnormalities are implanted in the uterus in hopes of achieving pregnancy.

Risks

Generally genetic tests have little physical risk. Blood and cheek swab tests have almost no risk. However, prenatal testing such as amniocentesis or chorionic villus sampling has a small risk of pregnancy loss (miscarriage).

Genetic testing can have emotional, social and financial risks as well. Discuss all risks and benefits of genetic testing with your doctor, a medical geneticist or a genetic counselor before you have a genetic test.

How You Prepare

Before you have genetic testing, gather as much information as you can about your family's medical history. Then, talk with your doctor or a genetic counselor about your personal and family medical history to better understand your risk. Ask questions and discuss any concerns about genetic testing at that meeting. Also, talk about your options, depending on the test results.

If you're being tested for a genetic disorder that runs in families, you may want to consider discussing your decision to have genetic testing with your family. Having these conversations before testing can give you a sense of how your family might respond to your test results and how it may affect them.

Not all health insurance policies pay for genetic testing. So, before you have a genetic test, check with your insurance provider to see what will be covered.

In the United States, the federal Genetic Information Nondiscrimination Act of 2008 (GINA) helps prevent health insurers or employers from discriminating against you based on test results. Under GINA, employment discrimination based on genetic risk also is illegal. However, this act does not cover life, long-term care or disability insurance. Most states offer additional protection.

What You Can Expect

Depending on the type of test, a sample of your blood, skin, amniotic fluid or other tissue will be collected and sent to a lab for analysis.

- **Blood sample**. A member of your health care team takes the sample by inserting a needle into a vein in your arm. For newborn screening tests, a blood sample is taken by pricking your baby's heel.
- **Cheek swab**. For some tests, a swab sample from the inside of your cheek is collected for genetic testing.

- **Amniocentesis**. In this prenatal genetic test, your doctor inserts a thin, hollow needle through your abdominal wall and into your uterus to collect a small amount of amniotic fluid for testing.
- **Chorionic villus sampling**. For this prenatal genetic test, your doctor takes a tissue sample from the placenta. Depending on your situation, the sample may be taken with a tube (catheter) through your cervix or through your abdominal wall and uterus using a thin needle.

Results

The amount of time it takes for you to receive your genetic test results depends on the type of test and your health care facility. Talk to your doctor, medical geneticist or genetic counselor before the test about when you can expect the results and have a discussion about them.

Positive Results

If the genetic test result is positive, that means the genetic change that was being tested for was detected. The steps you take after you receive a positive result will depend on the reason you had genetic testing.

If the purpose is to:

- **Diagnose a specific disease or condition**, a positive result will help you and your doctor determine the right treatment and management plan.

- **Find out if you are carrying a gene that could cause disease in your child**, and the test is positive, your doctor, medical geneticist or a genetic counselor can help you determine your child's risk of actually developing the disease. The test results can also provide information to consider as you and your partner make family planning decisions.

- **Determine if you might develop a certain disease**, a positive test doesn't necessarily mean you'll get that disorder. For example, having a breast cancer gene (BRCA1 or BRCA2) means you're at high risk of developing breast cancer at some point in your life, but it doesn't indicate with certainty that you'll get breast cancer. However, with some conditions, such as Huntington's disease, having the altered gene does indicate that the disease will eventually develop.

Talk to your doctor about what a positive result means for you. In some cases, you can make lifestyle changes that may reduce your risk of developing a disease, even if you have a gene that makes you more susceptible to a disorder. Results may also help you make choices related to treatment, family planning, careers and insurance coverage.

In addition, you may choose to participate in research or registries related to your genetic disorder or condition. These options may help you stay updated with new developments in prevention or treatment.

Negative Results

A negative result means a mutated gene was not detected by the test, which can be reassuring, but it's not a 100 percent guarantee that you don't have the disorder. The accuracy of genetic tests to detect mutated genes varies, depending on the condition being tested for and whether or not the gene mutation was previously identified in a family member.

Even if you don't have the mutated gene, that doesn't necessarily mean you'll never get the disease. For example, the majority of people who develop breast cancer don't have a breast cancer gene (BRCA1 or BRCA2). Also, genetic testing may not be able to detect all genetic defects.

Inconclusive Results

In some cases, a genetic test may not provide helpful information about the gene in question. Everyone has variations in the way genes appear, and often these variations don't affect your health. But sometimes it can be difficult to distinguish between a disease-causing gene and a harmless gene variation. These changes are called variants of uncertain significance. In these situations, follow-up testing or periodic reviews of the gene over time may be necessary.

Genetic Counseling

No matter what the results of your genetic testing, talk with your doctor, medical geneticist or genetic counselor about questions or concerns you may have. This will help you understand what the results mean for you and your family.

Telemedicine Robots

Excerpts from an mHEALTH-INTELLIGENCE article: Telemedicine Robots: Out of Science Fiction and Into the Mainstream
https://mhealthintelligence.com/features/can-telemedicine-robots-move-from-fantasy-to-fact

Originally designed to ferry supplies around the hospital or give surgeons a steadier hand for delicate medical procedures, robots are now finding their way into the care continuum, thanks to a variety of designs that can turn them into walking, talking healthcare kiosks. Healthcare robots can take orders from and deliver items to a patient, act as an around-the-clock sitter, assist frail and elderly patients out of a bed or chair, or provide a video connection to a distant doctor.

Robots have proven especially helpful in telemedicine. Companies like VGo and InTouch have developed robots that serve as the doctor's stand-in in remote clinics, community health centers, schools, cruise ships, sporting events, even smaller hospitals. They've even been used to provide home-bound or quarantine children with an avatar of sorts, enabling them to attend school and interact with classmates from afar.

Origins of Robots in Healthcare

Taking a page from the retail industry in the late 1990s, healthcare first turned to robots to automate the supply chain. Guided by GPS technology, small and squat mobile units were designed to deliver supplies, replacing the need to dispatch a nurse or other staff member to restock cabinets.

"This new robotic breed is boasting features increasingly found in smartphones, gaming consoles and other consumer electronics, from advanced sensors and motion detectors to powerful microprocessors and voice activation," the Wall Street Journal reported in 2012. "The service robots are self-aware, intelligent and able to navigate changing environments, even chaotic hospital settings."

Two types of robots are generally found in this environment: supply and maintenance robots such as the QC Bot and Aethon's Tugs robot, and mobile medical carts — often called computers-on-wheels or COWs. The latter are often dispatched to patient rooms to deliver patient orders or give doctors and nurses mobile access to medical instruments and the electronic medical record.

The first health systems to take full advantage of robots were pediatric hospitals that either ordered specially designed machines or dressed them up as characters to entertain their patients. More recently, these organizations used robots to help children adjust to the hospital and their care plan.

Many Different Uses for Robots

Robots are actually showing up in several healthcare scenarios. A blog in Medical Futurist outlines the nine most common uses:

1. <u>Room disinfection</u>. A robot using UV light can sterilize a room more effectively than housecleaning, reducing the chances of a hospital-acquired infection like MRSA or C.diff.

2. <u>Reception</u>. A robot can register patients, access medical records and provide detailed directions – in a y number of languages.

3. <u>Surgical assistance</u>. Robotic arms, guided by a doctor, can perform basic surgical procedures in small or delicate areas, even when the doctor is miles away.

4. <u>Remote clinical encounters</u>. Robots can serve as a doctor's eyes and ears in clinics, community centers, retail locations and the patient's home.

5. <u>Supply chain management</u>. Robots can carry up to 400 pounds of supplies from one department to another, be programmed to respond to shortages, even deliver food and amenities to patient rooms.

6. <u>Assisting mobility-impaired patients</u>. Some robots can assist patients getting in and out of beds or wheelchairs, while exoskeletons can improve mobility for patients with partial paralysis or other physical impairments.

7. <u>Drug delivery</u> (think Fantastic Voyage, without the human cargo). Miniaturized robots can be deployed inside the

body, delivering targeted doses of medication to specific locations, such as an organ or tumor.

8. <u>Blood drawing</u>. Newly developed robots can pinpoint the ideal vein and withdraw blood in half the time it takes a nurse to do the same thing.

9. <u>Patient engagement</u>. Robotic animals can help soothe the nerves of traumatized patients, especially children, or help them open up to care providers.

"As robots take care of our more intimate needs, such as personal caregiving, human to robot and robot to human interactions will become a central focus of study and philosophical discussion," healthcare IT blogger Bernadette Keefe, MD, wrote in a 2016 post for the Mayo Clinic.

"There is much unknown regarding the ultimate acceptability of robots in intimate settings, or at work," she concluded. "Comfort with robots may depend on multiple variables, such as the individual, culture, particular application, or industry. Trust is at the core of the use of autonomous robots in healthcare, and safety must be proven."

Related Article:

Smart Robotics for Smart Healthcare
https://lupinepublishers.com/robotics-mechanical-engineering-journal/pdf/ARME.MS.ID.000121.pdf

How to Start a Telemedicine Practice

Since I (the author of this book) am not familiar with the construction of a telemedicine business, I inserted the following articles from **Chiron Health, Inc**.

https://chironhealth.com/blog/how-to-start-a-telemedicine-practice/

New technology innovations have been changing the practice of medicine for many years. Digital medical records, electronic practice management systems, online patient portals, and other technologies allow physicians to operate more efficiently and reduce opportunities for error. Telemedicine is another advance that is capable of making practices more profitable, improving patient outcomes, and giving providers a new level of flexibility.

Conducting some visits remotely via video has excellent potential for practices. Starting a telemedicine practice may seem like a daunting task, but it is really quite easy if you follow some basic guidelines.

Before we talk about how to get started with telemedicine, let's chat a bit about why telehealth benefits practices.

Increased Revenue

Telemedicine visits are more efficient than in-person ones. This means that each provider can see more patients during the same amount of time. Because reimbursement for telemedicine is now widespread, practices can enjoy more revenue without the need to add providers, office staff, or office space.

Flexibility in Scheduling

Video visits can happen virtually anywhere, at any time. This gives practices the option to offer visits after hours or on weekends without requiring the physical office to be staffed.

Better Patient Outcomes

People are more likely to comply with recommendations for follow-up appointments if they don't have to come into the office. Telemedicine visits are also an effective way to increase patient engagement in medication management, chronic condition monitoring, and lifestyle coaching. Surveys show that patients are as satisfied, or even more satisfied with video visits.

Fewer No-Shows and Last-Minute Cancellations

No-shows and cancellations waste time and drain profits from medical practices. Setting up a telemedicine practice helps mitigate this problem by eliminating many of the factors that cause people to miss their appointments. The need to be at work, transportation issues, and lack of access to childcare don't become roadblocks when telemedicine is used. In fact, if a patient calls to say they can't make it into the office at the last minute, the visit can simply be switched to video.

Improved Work/Life Balance for Providers

Starting a telemedicine practice gives providers the option to work from home sometimes, or to see patients outside of traditional office hours. Many providers report that implementing a telemedicine practice helps them maintain a healthier work/life balance. For example, providers can connect with patients if needed even if they are away on vacation or traveling for business.

Protection from Competition

These days patients have many options besides a traditional medical office for care. Retail walk-in clinics and stand-alone urgent care centers are convenient ways for people to get on-demand care. At the same time, the number of options for online video visits continues to grow. Adding telehealth to a traditional practice is one way to protect against this type of competition.

Happier Employees

Healthcare providers love telemedicine, and the office staff does too. Telemedicine makes everyone more efficient by reducing the administrative tasks associated with an in-office visit. The waiting room is less crowded, and patients are happier. Video visits also lessen the potential for exposure to illness, and of course, all employees benefit from improved practice profitability.

Reimbursement for More Types of Visits

Another way that telehealth helps revenue growth is by turning something that providers often do for free today into paid activities. Most payers do not reimburse for telephone only follow-up visits, like reviewing test results or checking on the progress of a case. However, by using telemedicine to add a video component, these visits may become reimbursable.

If those are the kinds of practice improvements you are after, then it is time to think seriously about setting up your telemedicine practice. Here are the keys to success.

Select the Right Technology Partner

One of the most important decisions you will make when setting up a telemedicine practice is the technology that will power your remote visits. There are lots of options on the market, so it is critical to make a wise decision. To get started with telemedicine, look for a solution that meets the following guidelines:

Automated Reimbursement Verification

Telemedicine regulations vary by state, and insurance company payment policies also vary. The good news is that telemedicine is often reimbursed at the same rate as in-person visits. To be sure that you are paid for every video visit, find telemedicine technology that has built-in reimbursement verification. You'll be sure that you'll receive payment before the video visit is confirmed.

Integration with your EHR or Practice Management System

You don't want to have staff members duplicating information in multiple systems, so be sure that the telemedicine system you consider will integrate with your EHR or practice management solution. You should be able to seamlessly schedule appointments and send patient information between the systems securely.

Patient and Provider Support

Of course, you will look for telemedicine software that is easy to use, but there will be questions from time to time. Make sure that your technology partner will support your patients and your staff.

Scheduling

Consider solutions that handles scheduling in a way that works for your practice. Most providers prefer a solution that allows patients to request a video visit online, but gives actual control of the schedule to office staff.

Custom Branding

You want the process of setting up a telemedicine visit to be seamless for the patient and to support your brand. You can find a telemedicine system that lets you customize the look of the application to match your brand identity and include your logo.

The Ability to Work with Low Bandwidth and Slow Internet Connections

It is a best practice to use high-speed internet connections, but often medical office buildings have less than optimal networks. Be sure to find a solution that will work well in your environment.

HIPAA Compliance and Patient Privacy

The same requirements for patient privacy and information security that apply for in-person visits apply to visits conducted over video. When you start a telemedicine practice, you have the same responsibility to protect patient information. The storage of electronic files, video, and images must be approached with the same caution as you would take with physical documents.

Consumer-oriented services, like Skype and Facetime, do not support HIPAA compliant video conferencing because they are not encrypted. Therefore, they should never be used for any purpose that requires the use of Protected Health Information. Instead, look for telemedicine technology that has been designed to protect patient information.

Follow These Best Practices

Define the Goals for Your Telemedicine Program

It is smart to sit down and document the goals for your telemedicine program from the very beginning. Set clear goals with objective measurements. You include considerations like how you want your telehealth program to affect revenue, patient satisfaction, wait times, no-shows and cancellations, staff efficiency, retention, new patient acquisition, and any other metrics that are important for your practice.

Engage your Staff

Starting a telemedicine practice will have an impact on many functions within the practice, so it wise to get the right people involved in the roll-out of your program. We recommend putting together a task-force that includes providers who will be using telemedicine, staff members who will be scheduling appointments, and technical resources. When people get involved early and have the opportunity to help define the program, they become more invested in its success.

Study Reimbursement Rules and Regulations in Your State

State laws and payer policies about reimbursements for video visits vary widely. Most are becoming embracing telehealth because it is such an important tool for meeting the healthcare needs of the public. In fact, 31 states have what are known as "parity" laws, requiring reimbursement for telemedicine. But there is not a consistent national approach, so it is important to make yourself familiar with the regulations of your state.

Decide How Telemedicine Will Work Best for You

There is no one-size-fits-all strategy for leveraging telemedicine. You can craft an approach that meets the unique needs of your practice. Some providers block off specific times during the week for remote visits, while others decide to make video visits available during times that the office is traditionally closed. We mentioned the idea of conducting the follow-up phone calls that you already do using telemedicine to replace un-reimbursable telephone calls.

Work Hard to Make Patients Aware of the Option

It is critical to make sure that patients are aware that telehealth visits are an option for them. We recommend posting signs in the office, sending emails, and making a discussion about video visits part of every in-office encounter. Even if patients don't immediately schedule an appointment, knowing that telemedicine is an option may help keep them loyal to the practice despite increasing competition from retail health clinics and online-only providers. Some telemedicine technology providers even help market the service to patients on your behalf.

Ask for Feedback

When you first get started with telemedicine, it will be new to your staff and patients, so it is a great idea to gather their feedback. Find the best way for you to get the insight of both groups and integrate their best ideas into your telehealth program.

Check-In with Your Goals

Once you have launched your telemedicine practice, be sure to set up a periodic schedule for checking in with your goals. You may need to make tweaks to how you have implemented the approach. This is normal and to be expected. It is also smart to be sure to recognize and reward your team when you meet vital goals or milestones.

Starting a telemedicine practice is a big step, but it doesn't have to be a frightening one. If you find an excellent technology partner and stick to these best practices, you'll be reaping the benefits in no time.

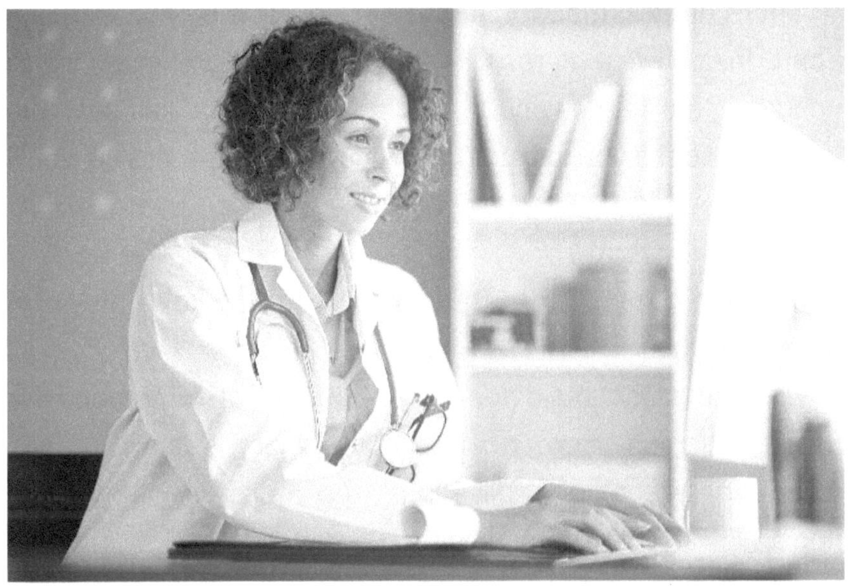

Essential Telemedicine Software Features

Article from **Chiron Health, Inc.**

https://chironhealth.com/blog/6-essential-telemedicine-software-features/

There are some features that most telemedicine systems have in common. Most support video conferencing with audio via the internet on the patient's PC or mobile device, for example. Vendors trying to sell you the lowest cost solution may argue that all telemedicine software is the same, but nothing could be further from the truth.

There are six important features that set the best solutions apart from the also-rans. These features are the key to ensuring that telemedicine is adopted and successful within your practice. If you insist on a solution that has them all, you'll be glad you did.

Support for Low Bandwidth and Slow Internet Connections

Medical office buildings and hospitals are infamous for having sluggish internet connections. At the same time, live video conferencing applications are notorious bandwidth hogs. Not a good combination. If the solution is slow or video quality is poor, your implementation will likely fail. That's why it is important to look for a telehealth solution that is designed to work well under less than optimal network conditions.

Full Patient and Provider Support

Some telehealth solutions, especially the very low-cost ones, offer very limited support for providers and no support at all for patients. In order for your telehealth program to be a hit with your staff and patients alike, choose a solution that will provide full, in-application support for your team and your patients.

Provider Scheduling

Some applications for video visits allow for patient-driven online appointment requests. This takes control of the telehealth program out of the hands of your staff. Provider scheduling, on the other hand, lets you decide when telemedicine appointments will be available.

Custom Practice Branding

You don't want your telehealth provider to come between you and your patients, potentially confusing them about who is providing their care. Choosing a solution that will include your brand identity helps providers and patients feel that telemedicine is an extension of your practice. You maintain a consistent brand across every type of interaction.

EHR Integration

Telemedicine solutions that integrate with your EHR system make your staff more efficient and reduce the opportunities for error. You can seamlessly schedule appointments and share patient information between systems.

Reimbursement Rules Engine

One of the reasons you are likely considering adding telemedicine to your practice is to increase revenue. Of course, you can't do that unless you are reimbursed for your video encounters. The complex landscape of state regulations and payer policies makes it difficult to be certain which patients are eligible for reimbursement. You and your team don't want to spend your valuable time becoming telehealth reimbursement experts. That's why you need a solution that will take the information about each patient, apply it against a sophisticated software algorithm, constantly updated by reimbursement experts, to determine if the patient is eligible.

(Full disclosure – We're the only solution provider that has one of these. We're so confident in its accuracy that we offer the industry's only Reimbursement Guarantee.)

Adding telemedicine to your practice is smart. Choosing a solution with these advanced features is smarter still. Doing so will greatly increase the likelihood that your program will be a success. Your patients and staff alike will thank you for it. (And so will your bottom line.) Interested in offering reimbursable video visits in your practice? Getting started with Chiron Health's user-friendly platform has never been easier!

Overcoming Roadblocks to Telemedicine Adoption

Article from **Chiron Health, Inc.**

https://chironhealth.com/blog/overcoming-roadblocks-telemedicine-adoption/

Recently Medscape, an online medical news resource, surveyed 1423 healthcare providers, including 847 physicians, and 1103 patients to assess their attitudes toward telemedicine and other emerging technologies in healthcare. The results show that while both providers and patients believe that technical advances can be used to improve patient health and increase access to care, they each have some reservations.

When it comes to telemedicine, patients and providers have a few overlapping concerns, but generally the roadblocks they see depend on their perspective in the doctor/patient relationship. The top concern for patients was getting the correct diagnosis. They also pointed to the lack of access to telemedicine as a big challenge. For providers, practice issues were top of mind, with malpractice and liability concerns ranking highest. Not surprisingly, reimbursement was also high on the list.

Every roadblock on the list is a legitimate area for concern. Fortunately, they can each be overcome by the right technology and some additional education. Let's have a look.

Top 4 Concerns for Physicians

Medical & Liability Concerns (60%)

While every provider should be sure that telemedicine is covered by their insurance policies, liability need not be a barrier to adopting a telemedicine program for a couple of reasons. First, telemedicine has been proven to be as effective as in-office encounters. In fact, more than 10,000 studies have been accepted by the National Library of Medicine supporting the clinical effectiveness and safety of telemedicine.

Next, malpractice claims related to telemedicine are rare. According to the risk management firm, WillisTowersWatson, "To date, there has been an almost infinitesimally small number of reported malpractice claims involving telemedicine. Even in those cases filed, telemedicine may not be the primary focus of the plaintiff's lawyer. Often, it is merely part of a fact pattern."

Reimbursement Concerns (43%)

Concerns about reimbursement are reasonable, but a combination of changing state laws and payer policies and new technology is making it easier for providers to put the reimbursement issue to rest. Twenty-nine states have laws on the books requiring that video visits be paid on par with in-office ones. Ten additional states are considering similar legislation.

In addition to the progressive movement in terms of legislation, modern telehealth technology solutions are stepping up to address the reimbursement issues as well. The Chiron Health solution includes our Rules Engine that validates the eligibility of a patient every time a remote visit is scheduled. Our Reimbursement Guarantee ensures that providers will get reimbursed for every verified encounter.

Technical Problems (40%)

Providers are also concerned about running into technical issues, such as poor audio and video quality due to low bandwidth connections. This can be addressed by ensuring that the network infrastructure is sufficient to support high definition video and choosing a telehealth solution that is designed to work in low bandwidth environments. Chiron Health, for example, requires just 10 Mbps download and 5 Mbps upload. You can test your speed at speedtest.net.

Privacy & Security Issues (40%)

Given the importance of HIPAA compliance, it's no wonder that privacy & security issues come up when providers think about telemedicine. Consumer video conferencing applications are not suitable for clinical encounters because they are not built for security. The good news is that there are purpose-built telemedicine applications that have HIPAA compliance backed in. There are also vendors that are happy to enter into business associate agreements with providers who use their solution.

Top 4 Concerns for Patients

Patient concerns mirror those of providers in some cases and differ in others. Here are the top five roadblocks patients see to implementing telemedicine:

Not Sure Diagnoses via Telemedicine are as Accurate (64%)

Overcoming this roadblock requires some education. As we mentioned above, hundreds of studies support the fact that telemedicine is as effective for diagnosing and treating many conditions as an in-person visit. Patients need reassurance that providers know which conditions can be effectively managed with telehealth and which require in-person evaluation.

My Physicians Don't Offer Telemedicine (51%)

Patients have a point with this one. Only 17% of the responding physicians in the Medscape survey reported seeing their own patients via telemedicine. This is a bit of a chicken-and-egg problem. Many physicians haven't considered telemedicine because their patients aren't asking for it, and patients aren't asking for it because they don't think that physicians offer it. However, the recent surge in the number of web-based healthcare companies that only offer telemedicine is starting to have an impact on the landscape as physicians realize that if they don't offer the convenience and cost savings of telehealth, their patients will seek it elsewhere.

Concerned About Insurance Coverage (40%)

This is the flip side of the reimbursement issue we discussed above. With advanced verification technology in place, providers can confidently assure patients that their validated visits will be covered.

Privacy & Security Issues (33%)

Of course, patients are concerned about keeping their health information confidential as well. Providers with HIPAA compliant software in place can reassure patients that their information is being adequately protected.

New technologies of any type always come along with a few barriers to adoption. When you are dealing with people's health, the need to be circumspect is even greater. But with the right information, careful thought, and well-designed technology they can be overcome.

Interested in offering video visits in your practice? Getting started with Chiron Health's simple user-friendly platform has never been easier!

Risk Management Issues and Strategies

Telemedicine: Risk Management Issues, Strategies and Resources

From the books and articles that I read, there have not been many reported telemedicine malpractice claims. This may be in part because the number of telemedicine visits, compared to in-person visits to a doctor, is still so low. Further, liability suits that have arisen may have been settled out of court and not reported. And even when claims are settled, confidentiality agreements could prevent any information from being disclosed.

It is not difficult to foresee liability issues as telemedicine grows in popularity. Therefore, I included the following article that highlights the risks of telemedicine.

I am an engineer - not a lawyer or healthcare expert. I wrote this book to provide information on the digital technology in telemedicine, but I realize that those directly involved in telemedicine need to understand the regulatory and liability issues surrounding it, and any coverage gaps that may exist with current professional liability policies.

A thorough understanding of the legal and regulatory issues associated with telemedicine is critical to successful deployment.

The following Article was originally printed in **Health Perspectives**.

Telemedicine is the practice of electronically connecting geographically discrete health care facilities and providers. It encompasses numerous methods and technologies, ranging from traditional store-and-forward data applications, commonly utilized in diagnostic review and interactive exams, to innovative "telepresent" methods, including robotic surgery and emergency services consultations. Among other uses, telemedicine applications permit:

- **Patients/clients in underserved rural areas** to enjoy improved access to quality care, and state-of-the-art settings.
- **Practitioner networks** to collaborate via shared electronic medical records, digital imagery and data files.
- **Specialty** providers to communicate with (or "tele-assist") primary care practitioners in diagnostic tasks, leading to enhanced outcomes, shorter treatment periods, decreased use of unnecessary drugs and reduced costs.
- **Emergency department personnel** to video-link with trauma specialists for instant access to life-saving information and support.

While telemedicine can foster efficiency and convenience, its reliance on continuous, real-time transmission of data over communication networks also creates risk. At every step of the process, adverse events may occur, including diagnostic errors, technical glitches, and patient/client privacy and security violations.

Healthcare Perspective outlines strategies designed to enhance clinical, operational and technical processes associated with the provision of telemedicine. National standards are cited throughout this resource, serving as policy templates in the following key areas: network security, confidentiality, quality improvement, informed consent, record maintenance and technical support.

Security

Safeguard patient/client data on computer networks and during transmission.

Secure transmission of clinical information requires effective safeguards at every point in the process, i. e., within the transmitting facility's network, over the transmission medium and at the distant site. Whether data are sent by satellite, through the Internet or over a virtual private network (VPN), the following security measures, among others, should be established and implemented:

Authentication enables authorized users to enter the system and access data via such means as log-in passwords, biometric scans, voice pattern samples and smart cards. Authentication procedures also permit system administrators to verify specific users and their means of interface. Outside access should be limited to those networks that fulfill organizational security requirements.

Patient/client identification uses patient/client integration profiles to promote accurate verification at multiple sites. These profiles enable the cross-referencing of patient/client identifiers either from multiple domains or from a central patient/client information server.

Data control ensures that patient/client information is stored and transmitted in a confidential manner through the creation of a VPN, use of encryption technology and/or file anonymization software. An increasing number of medical systems also require digital signatures to verify that data have not been modified by an unauthorized user. Encryption measures also should extend to stored data on portable devices or removable media, as theft and loss of laptops, tablets, smartphones, discs and USB flash drives are a leading source of data breaches.

Data tracking offers an audit trail of all exchanges involving medical information, permitting the system administrator to verify who has used the system and/or accessed patient/client data. Related monitoring technologies help identify and protect against technical glitches and hacking.

Protected access systems safeguard telemedicine applications on wireless networks. A variety of security mechanisms may be used to provide both logical and physical restrictions, including firewalls and antivirus software that detects malicious programs and activity.

Patient/Client Confidentiality

Privacy is a paramount concern when transmitting electronic data.

Unauthorized network access, hardware tampering and interception of data may violate privacy requirements imposed under HIPAA, as well as other governing federal and state laws and regulations.

Both telemedicine partners should implement a disclosure protocol incorporating the following practices:

- **Obtain written permission** (such as e-mail) from the patient/client before transmitting any protected health information.
- **Require all staff involved in telemedicine to execute confidentiality agreements**, including contract and vendor personnel.
- **Allow only designated professionals to disclose health related information**, such as the telepresenter and consulting and referring practitioners.
- **Mandate HIPAA training for staff and providers**, covering such topics as information security, common sources of breaches and consequences of protocol noncompliance.

- **Transmit patient/client data on an as-needed basis** and monitor staff for inappropriate access to protected health information.

The privacy obligations of health care practitioners extend to the environment where interactive consultations occur. The following provisions can help safeguard patient confidentiality:

- **Ensure that the patient/client is aware of and grants approval** for all personnel participating in consultations, including the telepresenter.
- **Place a conspicuous sign on the exam door**, notifying others that a consultation is in progress.
- **Prohibit the use of unauthorized cameras and cellular telephones in the examination room**, using a signed consent agreement if necessary.
- **Schedule telemedicine sessions in a designated area that is suitably enclosed and private**, rather than in an administrative suite or other public space.

Quality Improvement

Delivery of high-quality telemedicine services depends upon systematic monitoring and ongoing improvement of key processes. The following basic measures can help business owners more effectively compile, evaluate and report on meaningful care-related data.

Outcome measurement offers practitioners useful information about how well a telemedicine program is functioning, including further refinements that may be needed. Indicators should capture clinical, efficiency and satisfaction outcomes, including:

- Patient/client complication and morbidity rates.
- Compliance with provider performance criteria.
- Diagnostic accuracy.
- Adherence to clinical protocols.
- Referral rates.
- Patient/client satisfaction levels.
- Cost per case.
- Delays in accessing consultations, referrals or specialty providers.
- Average waiting times.

Standardized clinical protocols, properly implemented, can enhance quality and efficiency. By outlining a step-by-step process, protocols help improve consistency of care and performance of staff, and also ensure that test results are delivered in a timely, accurate and confidential manner. For interactive consultations, protocols minimally should advise providers on how and when to:

- Schedule a consultation.
- Arrange for a consulting room.
- Set up necessary equipment.

- Establish network connections.
- Prepare and advise the consulting provider, patient/client and telemedical presenter.
- Document consultation findings.
- Secure and back up required data.
- Prepare reports.
- Inform patients/clients and other providers of test results

The American Telemedicine Association has promulgated a variety of practice guidelines http://hub.americantelemed.orghttp://hub.americantelemed.org/resources/telemedicine-practice-guidelines

In addition, the Telehealth Resource Center provides information on protocol development www.telehealthresourcecenter.org/toolbox-module/creating-protocols

Incident reporting helps providers identify and respond to patient/client complications or other adverse events that may arise during telemedicine care. Providers should be instructed to document occurrences and forward reports promptly to the appropriate individual per written policy. A thorough, timely review of events helps foster a culture of accountability and continuous improvement.

Regular equipment testing and maintenance helps prevent potential technical and user problems. Equipment should be suitable for diagnostic and treatment uses, readily available when needed and fully functional during clinical encounters. Safety guidelines should specify who is responsible for maintenance. Utilize checklists or logs to facilitate documentation of post-installation testing, pre-session calibration, and ongoing quality checking of audio, video and data transmission capabilities.

Satisfaction surveys capture vital data regarding patient/clients and provider perceptions of the TMH program, as well as utilization patterns and the overall quality of TMH care. Surveys also can reveal unexpected barriers to care, including accessibility issues and cost.

Sample survey formats for telehealth encounters are available at https://healthit.ahrq.gov/sites/default/files/docs/survey/telehealthpatientsatisfactionsurvey_comp.pdf and www.techandaging.org/Telehealth_Patient_Satisfaction_Survey.pdf .

Training

Staff training should focus primarily on learning the skills necessary to conduct consultations and other TMH services smoothly and efficiently. At a minimum, training sessions should aim to enhance the following competencies:

- **Communication skills**, including video presentation content, organization and etiquette.

- **Understanding the scope of services** that can be provided using TMH methods.
- **Proficiency with the technology system in use**, as well as the physical environment.
- **Knowledge of operational protocols and procedures**, updated as necessary.
- **Ability to respond to equipment malfunctions** and manage unexpected occurrences.

Optimally, staff should begin with separate training sessions at the originating and distant sites, then progress to mock joint procedures before advancing to real-time provision of care. A wide variety of training modules is available, serving a range of procedures and existing proficiency levels. The Telehealth Resource Center offers guidance on developing a training strategy www.telehealthresourcecenter.org/toolbox-module/developing-training-strategy , as well as answers to commonly asked questions concerning training of TMH providers www.telehealthresourcecenter.org/toolbox-module/training .

Informed Consent

Patient/client consent is always required prior to participation in telemedicine services. Providers often use existing consent and documentation processes for store-and-forward consultations. For more invasive procedures, a separate consent form is preferable, encompassing the following information:

- Names, credentials, organizational affiliations and locations of the various health professionals involved.
- Name and description of the recommended procedure.
- Potential benefits and risks.
- Possible alternatives, including no treatment.
- Contingency plans in the event of a problem during the procedure.
- Explanation of how care is to be documented and accessed.
- Security, privacy and confidentiality measures to be employed.
- Names of those responsible for ongoing care.
- Risks of declining the treatment/service.
- Reiteration of the right to revoke consent or refuse treatment at any time.

In addition, clearly convey to the patient/client the inherent technical and operational hazards that may impede communication with the distant site or otherwise prevent prompt, accurate diagnosis of patient/client conditions. These include:

- **Communication line damage, satellite system compromise or other hardware failure**, which could lead to incomplete or failed transmission.
- **File corruption during the transmission process**, resulting in less than complete, clear or accurate reception of information or images.
- **Unauthorized third-party access**, which may lead to data integrity problems.
- **Natural disasters**, such as hurricanes, tornadoes and floods, which can potentially interrupt operations and compromise computer networks

Consent form documentation becomes part of the patient/client health care information record and is customarily maintained at the originating site, where the patient/client receives routine care.

Sample telemedicine informed consent forms are available from the American Telemedicine Association at https://thesource.americantelemed.org/resources/telemedicine-forms

Record Maintenance

Telemedicine sessions should be as thoroughly documented as all other patient/client encounters, with both partners to the telemedicine agreement contributing to the process. According to the American Health Information

Management Association, telemedicine records minimally should include:

- Patient/client name.
- Patient/client identification number at originating site.
- Date of service.
- Referring practitioner's name.
- Consulting practitioner's name.
- Provider organization's name.
- Type of evaluation to be performed.
- Informed consent documentation.
- Evaluation results.
- Diagnosis/impression of providers.
- Recommendations for further treatment.

The use of standardized intake and consultation forms can help providers achieve compliance with documentation parameters.

Templates, such as those available from the American Telemedicine Association, offer staff a clear and consistent documentation format for evaluations and consultations https://thesource.americantelemed.org/resources/telemedicine-forms .

Facilities also must select acceptable media for record keeping, such as electronic files, hard copy and/or video or audiotape. Protocol routinely dictates that the originating site retains files and images, providing the distant site with access to data when needed. Record retention policies should comply with professional standards, federal and state laws and regulations and the reimbursement requirements of public and private payers.

Health care business owners can help streamline the archiving process by assigning "lifespans" to patient/client data and medical documents stored in computer memories, based on such factors as last date of patient/client treatment, provider access requirements and record retention policies. For many organizations, data are maintained on a locally designated and protected server, with replication servers backing up files in the event of a disaster, computer problem or other type of business interruption.

Technical Support

Interactive telemedicine encounters depend upon a reliable and secure telecommunication system. Connections are of the utmost importance and should support business-grade videoconferencing with clear sound. Available options range from portable video conferencing units to large screen, high-definition consoles. Relying on the basic Internet for connection, rather than a private network dedicated to health care applications, may compromise quality and interfere with effective diagnosis or treatment.

Health care business owners can streamline the equipment selection process by compiling a list of general requirements and technical specifications for videoconferencing systems, ancillary devices and post-purchase support needs. Choices are generally guided by imaging needs, existing infrastructure and budgetary realities.

Regardless of the specific equipment selected, telemedicine systems should:

- **Comply with all relevant laws**, regulations and codes regarding patient/client safety and technical requirements.
- **Provide redundant systems** to help ensure uninterrupted network connectivity.
- **Utilize connections exclusively designated for telemedicine**, rather than local networks, which may be incompatible with telemedicine image transmission and archiving applications and/or lack sufficient bandwidth.
- **Permit networks to connect** through existing firewalls.

It also is necessary to accommodate the physical and environmental demands of telemedicine operations. Patient/client rooms must be sufficiently spacious to allow at least six feet between the patient/client and the camera operator. In addition, adequate HVAC capabilities and accessible infection control supplies – such as antibacterial wipes, sterile plastic sleeves for probes and camera lens disinfectant are essential to patient/client safety.

As with any new venture, successful implementation of a telemedicine program requires careful planning and collaboration by multiple stakeholders, both inside and outside the business. The strategies presented in this resource can help health care business owners initiate and maintain a high quality telemedicine program, which maximizes efficiency and convenience while minimizing associated risks.

https://www.wsna.org/news/2018/telemedicine-risk-management-issues-strategies-and-resources

Legal Notice

This article was originally printed in Health Perspectives. The content is based on the legal system of the USA.

The laws for telemedicine are different for each country.

2020 Telemedicine Trends (Edition II)

The world is globalizing. With information and technology expanding at a high rate, there are no signs of our advancements slowing down anytime soon. One of the industries that are taking advantage of this growth of technology and information is telemedicine.

Telemedicine is the essence of technology-driven healthcare and can serve as a lifeline for thousands if not millions of people who live in rural areas who do not have access to proper medical facilities.

The trend suggests however that remote patients won't be the only ones who benefit from telemedicine. An increasing number of patients who live in urban areas have also begun to take notice of this growing industry. This is because many people are interested in the convenience that telemedicine provides.

And, telemedicine doesn't just benefit the patient. It also benefits the provider. It allows providers to treat more patients simultaneously.

Telemedicine Trends

With the app culture so prevalent in our society, expect to see improved telemedicine apps that enhance communication between patient and provider. You can also expect to find apps that personalize your information that you can pull up with the swipe of a finger.

A rise in decentralized healthcare: In increasing numbers, healthcare professionals are migrating away from larger hospital complexes and opening up small community-based practices. This is a trend characterized by massive hospitals who offer their more specialized services in decentralized locations. It is predicted that younger healthcare professionals who prefer the flexibility that telemedicine offers will push for decentralization by opening the doors to their own telemedicine practices.

Stringent cyber security measures: Since telemedicine relies on technology, cyber security has become a necessity. With telemedicine becoming increasingly popular, information protection has become a top priority. We will likely see massive changes in the way the telemedicine industry goes about protecting confidential information.

Consolidation: Many smaller practices are struggling to keep their doors open. With the rise of business costs, stringent regulations, inability to expand properly and other factors, these small businesses have begun to look to other telemedicine companies for a solution. Some of these smaller operations will join up with larger telemedicine businesses who have the finances to thrive. These "coalitions" will allow bigger telemedicine operations to offer specialized services which they will acquire when they absorb failing practices. It's a win-win situation for everybody.

Proprietary hardware/software is becoming obsolete: For the most part, hospitals and the telemedicine industry have utilized proprietary software and hardware to offer their services to their patients. However, that may soon all change with the advent of easy to use secure software. Not only are these solutions user-friendly, but they are also far more affordable than implementing proprietary systems. Secure third party platforms will soon become the norm in the telemedicine industry.

Fewer trips to the emergency room: There's nothing you can do if you sprain your ankle. That will certainly require a trip to the emergency room. However, the ease and convenience of telemedicine make it easier to get treatable ailments looked at and diagnosed before it progresses to a point where a trip to the emergency room is required.

Millennial Appeal: The most relevant 2020 Telemedicine trend is the appeal to Millennials. As Millennials become the dominant patient base for many providers, the tools their practice utilizes must reflect the needs of their patients. Telemedicine appeals greatly to the millennial patient base due to its simplified nature and quick turnover. Patients can visit with their provider in a fraction of the time and then return to their busy lives. Partnered with a quality patient portal that allows them to view their information, pay their bills online, and communicate with their physician, this 2020 telemedicine trend appeals greatly to the millennial population.

The future for telemedicine looks bright

With more people becoming aware of telemedicine and its many options, the world will soon be taken by storm by this industry.

And, technologies such as low-latency 5G wireless capability and robotics are bringing innovation and cost reduction to healthcare. **5G wireless, in tandem with advances in artificial intelligence (AI) and edge computing architectures, will reduce healthcare costs while broadening access to more patients.**

Barriers to adoption of telemedicine

Yes, telemedicine has a great potential to improve access to care and ease the physician shortage. However, physician licensing, a lack of reimbursement parity laws and other legislation obstacles have hindered telemedicine's expansion.

The American Medical Association is however adding several new codes to its 2020 CPT code set to support remote patient monitoring and telehealth services. Among the 248 new codes added to the list for 2020, the AMA has created six for online digital evaluation services, or e-visits, in which care providers can connect with patients at home to exchange information.

Related Article:

2020 Healthcare Marketing Predictions:
https://healthcaresuccess.com/blog/healthcare-marketing/2020-healthcare-marketing-predictions.html

Closing Perspective

Although implementing telemedicine is complex and challenging, it is well worth the effort to bring care to patients who need a different type of healthcare setting. It has the potential of achieving better healthcare, lower costs, and improved public health - telemedicine can be a valuable tool.

However, remote monitoring can lead to additional strain on the networks in the healthcare industry. This increases congestion and slows network speeds. The lag is not only frustrating for those using it, but the poor quality can delay patient care, which could hurt outcomes in the long run. And because the use of Internet of Things (IoT) technologies continue to grow, the amount of data on networks is expected to increase. New technologies such as 5G and Wi-Fi 6 have the potential to help resolve these challenges. Broad availability of 5G is expected by 2025.

As technology continues to improve telemedicine will incorporate virtual reality, augmented reality, predictive data analytics, artificial intelligence and improved IT-technology such that anywhere someone has internet or cellular access, that person will also have access to medical care.

Despite the obstacles still in play, recognition that we need better health care options is vital to health care's future.
Telemedicine can be the Future of Healthcare!

Comments from health care professionals:

"Telemedicine will have far-reaching impacts on the current health care system that we can only begin to understand. While some are obviously good, such as lower costs for patients to access care, some will challenge hospitals and doctors to change their models to stay financially sound and relevant in the changing market. Laws and regulations will also have to change, and we can only hope that the laws change to enhance technological progress and increase access in health care while still protecting patients."

"In the future, connecting virtually with existing patients could be the norm. But hospitals are not technology experts. To deliver a seamless and friendly patient experience, they will need to engage with other companies. That is where telemedicine providers come in. They will have the technical expertise to develop sophisticated platforms that meet patient and provider needs."

"To really realize this vision of future telemedicine, at least two things need to happen. First, the technologies need to improve and become more stable. There will need to be rigorous testing to prove the concepts, especially if insurance is to reimburse any of the treatments or diagnostic tools. Second, physicians will need to be trained on the technologies and how to incorporate them into their practice."

www.ingramcontent.com/pod-product-compliance
Lightning Source LLC
Chambersburg PA
CBHW051439250726
48655CB00001B/143